The ADA Practical Guide to Dental Implants

Luigi O. Massa, DDS
Premier Dental Centers,
Art & Technology Dental Studio,
Boerne, TX, USA

J. Anthony von Fraunhofer, MSc, PhD, FADM, FRSC
Professor Emeritus, University of Maryland,
Baltimore, MD, USA

WILEY Blackwell   ADA American Dental Association®
America's leading advocate for oral health

This edition first published 2021
© 2021 by the American Dental Association

The right of Luigi O. Massa and J. Anthony von Fraunhofer to be identified as the authors of this work has been asserted in accordance with law.

Registered Office
John Wiley & Sons, Inc., 111 River Street, Hoboken, NJ 07030, USA

Editorial Office
111 River Street, Hoboken, NJ 07030, USA

For details of our global editorial offices, customer services, and more information about Wiley products visit us at www.wiley.com.

Wiley also publishes its books in a variety of electronic formats and by print-on-demand. Some content that appears in standard print versions of this book may not be available in other formats.

Library of Congress Cataloging-in-Publication Data

Names: Massa, Luigi O., author. | Von Fraunhofer, J. A. (Joseph Anthony),
    author. | American Dental Association, issuing body.
Title: The ADA practical guide to dental implants / Luigi O. Massa,
    J. Anthony von Fraunhofer.
Other titles: American Dental Association practical guide to dental
    implants | Practical guide series (American Dental Association)
Description: First edition. | Hoboken, NJ : Wiley-Blackwell, 2021. |
    Series: ADA practical guide | Includes bibliographical references and
    index.
Identifiers: LCCN 2021007918 (print) | LCCN 2021007919 (ebook) |
    ISBN 9781119630692 (paperback) | ISBN 9781119630661 (adobe pdf) |
    ISBN 9781119630685 (epub)
Subjects: MESH: Dental Implants
Classification: LCC RK667.I45 (print) | LCC RK667.I45 (ebook) | NLM WU
    640 | DDC 617.6/93–dc23
LC record available at https://lccn.loc.gov/2021007918
LC ebook record available at https://lccn.loc.gov/2021007919

Cover Design: Wiley
Cover Images: © Luigi O. Massa

Set in 9.5/12pt Palatino by SPi Global, Pondicherry, India

10 9 8 7 6 5 4 3 2 1

The ADA Practical Guide to Dental Implants

Table of Contents

Preface

Dentistry has a venerable history. Although prosthodontics has been practiced for several thousand years, the science of dentistry and dental care have made their greatest advances over the past 100+ years. What started out with the ground-breaking work of Greene Vardiman Black (1836–1915), reached its current extraordinary achievements and capabilities with a variety of innovations in the basic sciences, biomaterials science, radiography, dental armamentaria. . . and the dental implant.

The modern dental implant is based on the pioneering work of the Swedish orthopedic surgeon, Per-Ingvar Brånemark, in 1952.

Basically, a dental implant is a surgical fixture placed into the jawbone where it fuses with bone or osseointegrates over the span of a few months. Thus, the dental implant becomes a replacement for the root of a missing tooth such that it can support a replacement tooth or bridge. In fact, dental implants are now considered the standard of care for most prosthetic replacements of missing teeth.

The great advantage of an osseointegrated dental implant is that it is remarkably stable, mimics a natural tooth and will function independently of adjacent teeth. The success rate for dental implantology is now close to 98%, making dental implants the most successful of any restorative dental treatment.

This book was written in response to numerous requests to make available a practical guide to dental implants that functions as a virtual "how-to" manual for the dentist. What we have tried to do is discuss the many different aspects of dental implantology, even that difficult subject of economics, and give examples of each treatment modality covered in the text. We have also provided literature references so that the interested reader can delve more deeply into any subject that catches their interest.

We hope we have succeeded in our efforts and that this book will prove to be a useful guide and help to dentists as they embark upon the exciting task of placing and restoring dental implants for their patients.

Luigi O. Massa
New Braunfels, TX

J. Anthony von Fraunhofer
Boerne, TX

Why Dental Implants?

1

Why dental implants? There is one simple answer: there is an overwhelming need. Within the last one to two generations, there have been vast societal changes, including the fact that people are now living longer with greater motivation to maintain the function and esthetics of their natural teeth. It was common for people just 60 or so years ago to lose most, if not all, of their teeth well before retirement age. As a result, dentistry prior to the 1960s was largely focused on providing restorations for carious teeth and fabricating removable appliances such as removable partial dentures (RPDs) and complete dentures (CDs) as the final dental solutions for missing teeth.

Partial and Complete Edentulism in the Twenty-First Century

The population is aging and, by 2030, more that 20% of the U. S. population will be aged 65 years or older, Fig. 1.1 [1].

These projected data indicate that within 10–12 years, about 20% of the population will be "senior citizens," namely 65 years or older [1]. Although advances in medicine and pharmacology, together with improved nutrition, dietary awareness and exercise, have significantly improved the average life expectancy, the outlook for maintained and even improved dental hygiene as well as overall oral health still looks bleak. In fact, partial or complete edentulism is increasing. Whereas fluoridation has markedly reduced dental caries [2, 3], the prevalence of tooth loss through periodontal disease, enamel erosion, wear, trauma and disease (e.g., cancer) is growing [4–7].

The ADA Practical Guide to Dental Implants, First Edition. Luigi O. Massa and J. Anthony von Fraunhofer.
© 2021 The American Dental Association. Published 2021 by John Wiley & Sons, Inc.

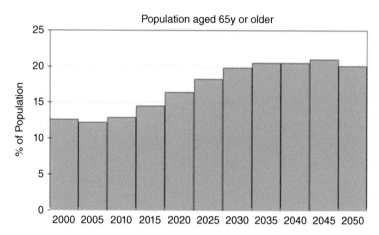

Figure 1.1 Projected aging of the United States. (*Source*: Based on United States Census Bureau. Release Number CB20-99: 65 and Older Population Grows Rapidly as Baby Boomers Age. Washington, DC, June 25, 2020).

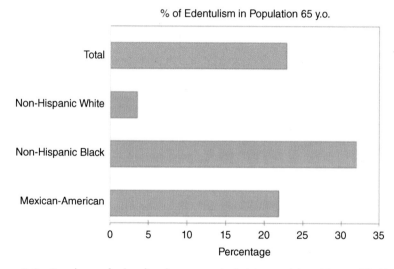

Figure 1.2 Prevalence of edentulism by race and ethnicity in adults ≥65 years [9]. (*Source*: Based on Centers for Disease Control and Prevention. Edentulism and tooth retention. Atlanta, Ga., September 10, 2019).

According to the American College of Prosthodontics, more than 35 million Americans are edentulous, and 178 million people are missing at least one tooth and these numbers are expected to grow over the next two decades [8].

What is distressing about these statistics is that edentulism affects our most vulnerable populations – the aging and the economically disadvantaged, Fig. 1.2. In the geriatric population, for example, the ratio of edentulous to dentate individuals is 2 : 1, with about 23 million being completely edentulous and some 12 million are edentulous in one arch. About 90% of edentulous patients have dentures and some 15% of edentulous patients will have dentures made each year [8].

The consequences of partial or complete edentulism are well-known and include many facets of the quality of life (QoL) as well as facial appearance, self-image and self-confidence. Overall, health consequences of edentulism encompass significant nutritional changes, digestive issues, obesity, diabetes, and coronary artery disease to name but a few.

The Reality of Dental Implants

Although there have been minor variations over the past few years, the current life expectancy for the U.S. population in 2020 is 78.93 years [10], and we can anticipate increases in tooth failures. Vertical root fractures, endodontic failures, restorative failures, and periodontal disease may result in tooth loss. In contrast to the practice of dentistry in the nineteenth and twentieth centuries, modern dentistry focuses on the replacement of lost teeth utilizing implants, combined with comprehensive analysis of function and esthetics.

In modern dentistry, the dental implant is the best tooth replacement option for nearly all situations where a tooth is missing or is failing. The primary reason for this is the extremely high success rate achieved with dental implants. Saving teeth at all costs is no longer the norm because of the unpredictability of the longevity of heroic dentistry. In other words, preserving bone and tissue regeneration are now considered to be more important than trying to prolong tooth retention. This approach not only promotes bone healing and preservation but ensures that implants are placed in a predictable and solid bony environment with a high rate of success.

The consensus regarding dental implants within the international dental community can be summarized in Table 1.1. Whereas the order of the comments may vary with the individual clinician, most would agree that these comments are valid and pertinent.

Implants and the Edentulous Patient

Over 32 million people in the U.S. wear partial or CDs [11] and approximately 33% of these patients complain that their dentures fit poorly, tend to loosen or dislodge during activities such as chewing and laughing, and/or there is pain on mastication. Flat ridges and/or shallow palatal vaults add to denture retention and instability problems and most dentists are aware that the mandibular CD presents retention issues.

Table 1.1 Advantages of dental implants.

- Implant dentistry is the future of dentistry.
- There is copious scientific literature on dental implantology.
- The 95–97% success rate of dental implants makes them an extremely predictable treatment.
- There is an overwhelming need for tooth replacement and predictable treatment of failing teeth.
- Implant-retained prosthetics are a very satisfactory solution to the growing prevalence of edentulism in our aging population.

Limitations and/or restrictions on diet, especially which foods can or cannot be eaten, also play a major role in the decision to seek dental implants. It is likely that a significant percentage of those patients experiencing pain or discomfort on chewing will not use their dentures during eating. Due to the decreased mastication forces associated with dentures, edentulous patients have been found to consume less food and have lower intakes of protein, intrinsic and milk sugars, non-starch polysaccharides (fibrous matter), calcium, non-heme iron, niacin and vitamin C than dentate people [12]. These dietary deficiencies often have significant adverse effects on overall health and wellbeing, as well as their QoL.

Many patients will resort to utilizing denture adhesives to aid in retention. These adhesives may lead to further problems as they are extremely difficult to remove from the tissues. Impaired speech patterns as well as halitosis (oral malodor or "denture breath") are frequent complaints among denture wearers, even when the fit of the denture is not a significant issue.

It follows from the above, that patients seek dental implant therapy for a number of reasons, including the following:

• Function
• Esthetics
• Comfort
• Confidence
• Facial appearance

General dental practitioners can address these issues and assist the patient in achieving oral health and functionality lost through missing teeth.

There are two major implant treatment modalities for the edentulous patient:

1. Implant over-dentures. Implant overdentures are removable appliances which are both implant and tissue-borne prostheses. They utilize an abutment and a denture attachment for the retention (Fig. 1.3). These appliances solve several major problems with traditional dentures by allowing:
   • Increased masticatory forces
   • Increased retention to potentially eliminate the need for denture adhesives
   • Removal of palatal coverage for patients who cannot tolerate the denture due to their gag reflex
   An implant-supported denture is a satisfactory and viable economic alternative to the traditional CD.
   • Screw-retained fixed implant bridges. Fixed implant bridges are implant-borne prostheses which are not removable by the patient. They are manufactured in zirconia or in acrylic overlaying a chrome-cobalt or titanium bar. These appliances give patients the greatest masticatory forces and are more appealing to most patients because they are fixed in place.

Implants for Single Crowns and Bridgework

As stated above, 178 million people in the U.S. are missing at least one tooth [11]. Before the use of dental implants, fixed partial dentures (bridges) or RPDs were utilized. One major problem with these treatment modalities is that fewer teeth

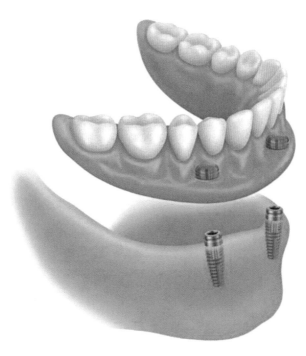

Figure 1.3 Implant-supported overdenture. *Source*: Courtesy of Zest Anchor.

are taking the load. For example, in the case of a four-unit fixed bridge, only two teeth are carrying the load of the four teeth it restores because the pontics provide no functional support.

The advantages for placing an implant and restoring it to replace a missing, free-standing tooth are summarized in Table 1.2.

Table 1.2 Advantages of implants replacing individual teeth.

No unnecessary preparation of adjacent teeth for a traditional bridge
Long-term prognosis better than for a traditional bridge [13, 14]
Long-term cost is less than for a traditional bridge
Significantly better retention of prostheses, including RPD's
In the authors' opinion, ease of dental hygiene is improved with implants as opposed to a
traditional bridge
Greater long-term patient satisfaction

Dentists are accustomed to replacing multiple missing teeth with a RPD. In fact, RPDs have been a viable treatment option for decades. While they serve a recognizable and useful purpose, they do require some skill and much experience in regard to their design and fabrication.

Despite their many advantages, which include relatively low cost, RPDs have some major drawbacks. In particular, they can lead to increased ridge resorption, especially with appliances fabricated with non-metallic bases, i.e., what are commonly known as "flippers."

Whereas RPDs with polymeric (usually acrylic) clasps are somewhat "kinder" to supporting teeth, metallic clasps and rests will commonly traumatize the clasped teeth over time, notably causing wear and abrasion. This destructive action is due to clasps riding up and down the anchor teeth due to flexure of the RPD during mastication or parafunctional activities. Poor fit and/or repetitive vertical (and lateral) movements due to cyclic loading will not only exacerbate wear and abrasion of the abutment teeth but increase ridge resorption.

Another problem with RPDs, especially those with polymeric bases and poorly-fitting appliances, is that food particles may often be trapped beneath the denture. This can lead to mucosal irritation, periodontal problems and, possibly, to decay of the supporting teeth. Further, staining of the acrylic "gum work" of the RPD as well as odor necessitates repeated and careful cleaning of the RPD on at least a daily basis to ensure a hygienic appliance and absence of halitosis. Depending upon diet and beverage consumption as well as smoking, there is often the need for more frequent cleaning of the RPD. Failure to remove the RPD and clean teeth and RPD separately compromises effective hygiene of both teeth and RPD.

There are, of course, some disadvantages to the use of implants to replace multiple teeth, Table 1.3.

Table 1.3 Disadvantages of implants vs traditional bridgework and RPDs.

Short-term cost is higher than for a traditional bridge or RPD
Surgery is required
Generally, treatment time is longer – 4–8 months.

Implants vs Endodontic Treatment

Although general dentists receive training in endodontics during their education, many prefer not to provide root canal therapy, particularly when surgical intervention is required. There are several reasons for this reluctance to perform surgical endodontics, not the least is the general perception of patients that "root canal therapy" is an unpleasant, long-drawn out procedure that can be uncomfortable at best and at worst is painful. In fact, to a great many patients, the words "root canal therapy" are synonymous with any procedure or experience that is to be avoided at almost any cost.

In contrast, non-surgical endodontic treatment is a predictable treatment choice if certain conditions are met. First, there must remain enough sound tooth structure to achieve a 2mm ferrule effect 360° around the tooth. This will ensure long-term stability of restorative treatments. Secondly, a cause-and-effect should be established when diagnosing a symptomatic tooth. For example, caries approximating a pulp horn with symptoms lead to a clear diagnosis of irreversible pulpitis. Conversely, a symptomatic tooth with no caries present leads to a less predictable treatment outcome until and unless a definitive diagnosis can be achieved.

When there is need for "root canal therapy," the operator must have available a specialized armamentarium of instruments and restorative materials. However, it must be stated that the available instrumentation and endodontic sealer cements have improved dramatically over the past 20 or so years. Further, it is generally recognized that the time and expertise required to perform endodontic surgery increases almost exponentially with the number of tooth roots/canals to be treated. Additionally, when canals are sclerosed or calcified, there is increased difficulty in ensuring a clean and extirpated pulpal chamber and root canals.

Finally, teeth that have received extensive endodontic therapy tend to embrittle over time and are subject to failure under loading. Further, it is difficult to achieve a complete hermetic seal of a root canal so that apical leakage and ingress of bacteria, blood and other matter into the treated canal can occur over time. Coronal migration of tissue fluids and bacteria leaking into the treated root canal over time can have many untoward consequences, including dentinal staining, breakdown of sealer cements and restorations, pain and discomfort as well as infection. Due to risks associated with endodontically treated teeth, dentists are often reluctant to use these teeth as abutments for both FPDs and RPDs.

In contrast, the success rate of dental implants is 95–97%. This is far higher than treatment of symptomatic teeth with marginal ridge fractures and endodontic retreatment. These success rates must be considered when discussing treatment options, particularly when relative costs, patient time-commitment to treatment as well as patient discomfort are considered in addressing the question of root canal therapy vs placement of an implant.

Conclusions

Having presented the overall case for dental implants, specific factors regarding the placement and clinical application of implants will be covered in detail in the following chapters. Nevertheless, modern dentistry now recognizes that dental implants are the standard of care for prosthetic replacement of missing teeth. This is because they can readily and conveniently address some otherwise seemingly intractable problems in traditional restorative dentistry. Further, the advances in implant technology and dental science have progressed so markedly since the first days of the Brånemark concept that the outcome of dental implant placement has a success rate over 95%.

The final word should be that the ground-breaking concept of Per-Ingvar Brånemark has transformed dentistry and dental treatment for even the most challenging cases.

References

1. United States Census Bureau (2020). 65 and Older Population Grows Rapidly as Baby Boomers Age. Release Number CB20-99. https://www.census.gov/newsroom/press-releases/2020/65-older-population-grows.html (accessed 17 December 2020).
2. Medjedovic, E., Medjedovic, S., Deljo, D. et al. (2015). Impact of fluoride on dental health quality. *Mater. Sociomed.* 27 (6): 395–398.
3. Centers for Disease Control and Prevention (2001). Recommendations for using fluoride to prevent and control dental caries in the United States. *MMWR Recomm. Rep.* 50 (RR-14): 1–42.
4. Martinez-Canut, P. (2015). Predictors of tooth loss due to periodontal disease in patients following long-term periodontal maintenance. *J. Clin. Periodontol.* 42 (12): 1115–1125.
5. Loomansa, B., Opdamb, N., Attinc, T. et al. (2017). Severe tooth wear: European consensus statement on management guidelines. *J. Adhes. Dent.* 19: 111–119.

6. Bartlett, D.A. (2005). The role of erosion in tooth wear: etiology, prevention and management. *Int. Dent. J.* 55: 277–284.

7. Michaud, D.S., Fu, Z., Jian Shi, J. et al. (2017). Periodontal disease, tooth loss, and cancer risk. *Epidemiol. Rev.* 39 (1): 49–58.

8. American College of Prosthodontists (2020). Facts and figures. https://www.gotoapro.org/facts-figures (accessed 31 July 2020).

9. Centers for Disease Control and Prevention (2019). Edentulism and tooth retention. September 10. https://www.cdc.gov/oralhealth/publications/OHSR-2019-edentulism-tooth-retention.html (accessed 27 December 2020).

10. Macrotrends (2020). U.S. Life Expectancy 1950–2020. https://www.macrotrends.net/countries/USA/united-states/life-expectancy (accessed 31 July 2020).

11. Statista Research Department (2020). Usage of dentures in the U.S. http://www.statista.com/statistics/275484/us-households-usage-of-dentures (accessed 31 July 2020).

12. Jauhiainen, L., Männistö, S., Ylöstalo, P. et al. (2017). Food consumption and nutrient intake in relation to denture use in 55- to 84-year-old men and women — results of a population based survey. *J. Nutr. Health Aging* 21: 492–500.

13. Ravidà, A., Tattan, M., Askar, H. et al. (2019). Comparison of three different types of implant-supported fixed dental prostheses: a long-term retrospective study of clinical outcomes and cost-effectiveness. *Clin. Oral Implants Res.* 30 (4): 295–305.

14. Oh, S.-H., Kim, Y., Park, J.-Y. et al. (2016). Comparison of fixed implant-supported prostheses, removable implant-supported prostheses, and complete dentures: patient satisfaction and oral health-related quality of life. *Clin. Oral Implants Res.* 27 (2): e31–e37.

A Brief History of Dental Implants 2

Dentistry has a venerable history in that prosthodontics has been practiced for several thousand years. Fine examples of dental bridgework dating from around 700 BCE were crafted by the Etruscans of Central Italy (now Tuscany) and fixed partial dentures are known to have been fabricated by the Maya of Central America as far back as 700 CE [1–4]. There are many well-known figures in history, for example, Queen Elizabeth I of England, King Henry II of France, George Washington of the United States and Winston Churchill of the United Kingdom, all of whom either wore removable partial dentures (RPDs) or complete dentures (CDs) [3].

The "father" of dentistry is generally acknowledged to be the French physician Pierre Fauchard (1678–1761) [2] whereas most historians and dentists credit Dr. Greene Vardiman Black (1836–1915) [2, 5, 6] as the "father of modern dentistry." There are a number of other pioneers in dentistry, including the illustrious Scottish surgeon John Hunter, an early advocate of careful observation and scientific observation in medicine. Not only did Hunter collaborate with his former student Edward Jenner, the pioneer of the smallpox vaccine, but he also dabbled (unsuccessfully) with transplanting teeth, possibly following on from the work of Ambroise Paré (1510–1590). Paré is recognized as the "Father of Modern Surgery" and, interestingly, as the "Foster Father of Dental Surgery." Interestingly, Paré referred to transplanting of teeth as early as 1564.

Despite its venerable history, the greatest advances in dentistry have really only occurred within the latter half of the twentieth century and, notably, the past 50–60 years. Many influences have transformed dentistry from an ancient quasi-craft into the evidence-based technological science it is today, including the innovative work of early dental practitioners, advances in oral medicine, oral surgery and restorative dental techniques, together with an astonishing array of

The ADA Practical Guide to Dental Implants, First Edition. Luigi O. Massa and J. Anthony von Fraunhofer.
© 2021 The American Dental Association. Published 2021 by John Wiley & Sons, Inc.

Table 2.1 Innovations in dentistry and dental care.

Acrylic resin
Adhesive dentistry
Air-turbine handpieces
Bowen's resin
Computer-aided designed/computer-aided manufactured restorations
Chromium-cobalt casting alloys
Composite restorative materials
Cosmetic dentistry
Dental Amalgam
Digital radiography
Direct bonding of orthodontic brackets
Electric high-torque/high-speed handpieces
Endodontic therapy
Endosseous oral implants
Fluoride-containing dentifrices
Glass ionomers
High-strength dental ceramics
Mechanical toothbrushes
Orthognathic surgery
Porcelain fused to metal restorations
Silver-palladium alloys
Visible light-cured restorative materials
Water fluoridation

scientific and technology-driven progress in dental science and dental biomaterials. Table 2.1 indicates a significant number of innovations that have changed modern dentistry, one of which is the endosseous dental implant.

The confluence of the advances in the basic sciences, dental biomaterials and clinical technique possibly reached their apex in the endosseous dental implant, perhaps the most successful dental restorative technique ever devised. Virtually no other dental procedure has achieved the long-term success rate found over the past 15–20 years with dental implants.

Replacing Missing Teeth

The efforts of Ambroise Paré, John Hunter and others to replace missing teeth through implantation of sound teeth from donors were the initial attempts to address this need in patients. Dentures, as such, were not available for the general populace back in the fifteenth and sixteenth centuries and only the very wealthy could avail themselves of transplanted teeth or the rudimentary dentures of that period. Charles Allen of York, England, the author of the first English book solely on dentistry [7] was very dismissive of tooth transplantation.

Patients seemed to accept the limited durability of transplanted teeth and transplantation, probably due to clever publicity and hucksterism, became almost a craze on the European Continent, in England and even America in the late eighteenth century. Sadly, through the sixteenth, seventeenth, and eighteenth centuries, paupers often sold their teeth for cash to earn a little money and the heroine Fantine in Victor Hugo's *Les Misérables* (1852) was forced to sell her hair, then her incisors and finally her "virtue" in order to survive. Despite its lack of success and almost total disregard of the basic precepts of oral hygiene, tooth transplanting continued well into the nineteenth century. In fact, barrels of teeth extracted from casualties in the American Civil War were regularly shipped to England, and presumably Europe, for both transplantation and to be used in constructing dentures.

This situation changed with the advent of dental schools, the establishment of professional standards and the growing awareness of the general public that dentistry, dental care and oral hygiene were important not only to the oral cavity but also to systemic health. Nevertheless, despite the venerable history of dentures and the remarkable success of modern CDs, FPDs, and RPDs, many patients simply do not like the fact that they must resort to prostheses to preserve masticatory efficiency and maintain facial esthetics. As any dental professional recognizes, there are myriad reasons that patients complain about their dentures. Many complaints, arising from poor denture fit, discomfort, inadequate retention and even pain, are completely understandable and often justified whereas others arise from a basic dislike of a "foreign body" in the mouth. Further, the need for careful oral hygiene and meticulous cleaning of removable appliances is commonly viewed as an unwelcome chore if not an imposition. The perception of many patients is that all of these factors, combined with many others, contribute to the steadily growing appeal of a dental implant that appears to be permanent, painless, and "maintenance-free."

Dental Implants

A major problem with CDs, especially for the mandible, is poor retention, often exacerbated by residual alveolar bone above basal cortical bone. Resilient linings, denture creams and other retention aids may alleviate the problem on a temporary basis but rarely "cure" retention or stability issues. One approach to addressing such concerns during the 1970s and, subsequently, was the subperiosteal implant which comprised a metallic framework that closely fit and sat directly on the bone of the mandible.

Subperiosteal Implants

The basic concept of the subperiosteal implant was that a CD rested on abutments that projected through the mucosa, Fig. 2.1. Consequently, masticatory and other stresses were transmitted directly to the supporting bone rather than to the oral mucosa as with conventional CDs. This approach enabled the surgeon to trim the basal bone of any projections or spicules of residual bone to ensure a good fit for the framework but also, incidentally, could help reduce or eliminate any painful sore spots for the final CD.

Fabricating a subperiosteal implant, however, was a long and rather involved procedure. The mandibular mucosa had to be reflected and an impression made of the exposed bone. A wax pattern was then designed on the gypsum cast and used as the pattern for a chrome-cobalt cast framework. In a subsequent procedure, the mucosa was reflected again, and the framework placed on the exposed bone before the mucosa was restored in position and healing allowed to

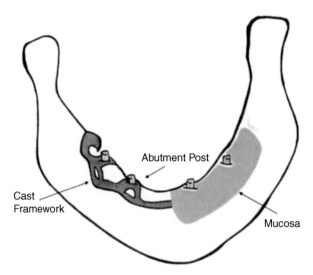

Figure 2.1   The subperiosteal implant.

start. After healing, a CD could be fabricated and seated on the abutments projecting through the mucosa. There were three principal varieties of subperiosteal implant: full mandibular, full maxillary, and unilateral or single-unit implants. The latter were smaller than full arch implants and had only one protruding abutment. They were particularly useful when used as terminal abutments for edentulous quadrants, i.e., free-end saddle retention aids.

Although subperiosteal implants were effective, the overall procedure was lengthy and involved a great deal of discomfort for the patient and often were subject to various complications [8, 9]. Further, a high degree of surgical skill was required and necessitated a close collaboration between the surgeon, prosthodontist, and the laboratory technician to ensure optimal clinical results. Provided care was exercised in patient selection, there was good overlying soft tissue and no residual alveolar bone, the prognosis could be very good with reasonably high short-term success rates.

Endodontic Implants

For many years, the most established and longest established implant was the endodontic endosseous pin implant, also known as the endodontic stabilizer, and was particularly useful for rigidly anchoring a mobile tooth to bone. Tooth mobility can have many causes, including an unfavorable crown-to-root ratio, gum and alveolar recession, bruxism and an unbalanced occlusion.

The basis of this approach was that a pin was inserted through the root canal into the underlying bone such that it was anchored in bone but with upper end projecting into the mouth and upon which, a crown or RPD was fabricated [10].

Typically, the lower end of the pin did not penetrate the cortical plate of the mandible or the antral or nasal floors of the maxilla. Indications for endodontic implants included treatment of root fractures, external or internal root resorption and when better support and stability was required for FPD or RPD abutments.

Although the clinical use of endodontic endosseous pin implants is less common due to the advent of the modern endosseous implant, they were successful, with few contraindications for their use provided correct clinical procedures were followed [11].

Endosseous Implants

Endosseous implants, also known as intra-osseous and endosteal implants, have been in clinical use since the 1960s [12]. There are four main categories of endosseous implant, namely pins, spirals, blades, and screws. Regardless of implant design, endosseous implants are used in edentulous areas where there is sufficient healthy bone to accommodate the implant. Selection criteria for the use of implants are discussed in later chapters of this book.

The first successful endosseous implants were the Formiggini spiral screw implant and, subsequently, the Cherchève spiral-post implant, the former dating from 1947 and the latter from the 1960s to 1970 [4, 12]. The most sophisticated, and successful, Cherchève implant consisted of a double hollow spiral mounted on a square post. After the bone was trephined to create a cavity, the implant was placed beneath the alveolar ridge with the shank or post extending into the oral cavity and, upon which, the final prosthesis was constructed. The problem with these early implants was that trephining of the bone created a gap or space between the abutment post and the host hard and soft tissues, and this could sometimes present problems.

Many workers developed modifications of the spiral implant during the late 1960s and early 1970s. These largely comprised self-tapping screw implants, often with a vent or port below the threaded portion to permit fibrous tissues and, hopefully, bone to grow through the aperture and promote retention. Although many of these screw implants were successful, numerous failures occurred as the result of tissue irritation, frank infection and epithelial downgrowth preventing adequate retention and sometimes complete evulsion of the implant. Commonly, poor bony attachment to these implants caused stability to be a problem.

An alternative approach to screw-type endosseous implants was the tripodal pin concept which dated from the same period. In essence, thin tantalum pins were inserted into bone at roughly 120° angulations and the exposed ends of the pins were bonded together using acrylic resin, Fig. 2.2.

The implanted tripodal system could then be used as a bridge abutment or to support a single-unit prosthesis. Although pin implants had certain applications, they did not possess long-term retention, generally were not self-supporting and the pins often were easily displaced or removed over time.

A major development in endosseous implants was the blade or blade vent implant designed by Linkow in 1968 and subsequently modified by Linkow and others over the period 1970–1971 [12–14]. Blade implants were originally designed for use in areas where there were knife-edge alveolar ridges, situations where screw-type implants are contra-indicated. These implants can be used in virtually all maxillary and mandibular edentulous areas, provided there is sufficient residual alveolar process. Because the implants have greater mesio-distal dimensions than their vertical heights, the design combines maximal

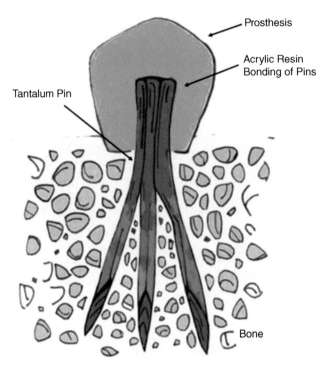

Prosthesis

Acrylic Resin
Bonding of Pins

Tantalum Pin

Bone

Figure 2.2 Schematic diagram of tripodal pin concept.

stability, especially against lateral forces, while minimizing risk to underlying tissues and structures.

Clinically, bone often grew through the vents of the blade implants so that the early success rate was very high although the long-term prognosis was lower, especially with maxillary placements. Various problems were associated with blade implants, particularly the difficulty in achieving an ideal gingival relationship with that crown when used to support a single crown. There were also problems with thin ridges such that any bony destruction could result in implant loss. Apparently, fewer problems were found with blades used to support a denture base although stability was a problem with unilateral mandibular free-end saddles.

The modern "screw" implant derives from the pioneering work of Stefano Tramonte [15] in Italy and Per-Ingvar Brånemark in Sweden [16, 17], both of whom advocated the use of titanium for dental implants.

The excellent physical properties and outstanding biocompatibility of titanium were the driving force for this application. In particular, Brånemark described the clinically observed close apposition and adherence of bone with titanium, which he termed osseointegration. Since then, a wide variety of "screw" or tooth root-shaped endosseous implants have come into clinical use, Fig. 2.3 and Fig. 2.4 and they have achieved remarkable clinical success such that they are now considered important components of the restorative dentistry armamentarium. However, the clinical success of dental implants requires good clinical technique, accurate placement and careful patient selection with good bone quality (see later chapters in this book).

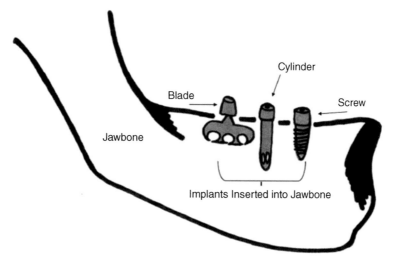

Figure 2.3   Different types of implants.

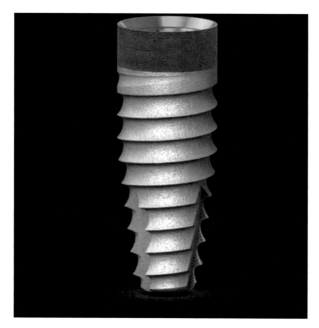

Figure 2.4   Modern screw-type implant. (*Source*: Courtesy of Biohorizons).

Of central importance for any metal within the oral cavity is corrosion resistance as well as mechanical strength. Consequently, the vast majority of modern dental implants are fabricated from titanium and its alloys, notably Ti-6Al-4V, the so-called 6-4 alloy, although CP (commercial purity) Titanium and alloys such as Ti-13Cu-4.5Ni have also been evaluated. Most implants are fabricated using powder metallurgy, typically hot isostatic pressing HIP technology.

The efficacy and rate of osseointegration of bone and implant has been enhanced by techniques such as designing the implant with a screw profile, providing a micro-texture to the implant surface as well as coating the surface with hydroxyapatite (HA). More recently, a novel approach to dental implantology has been to coat the implant surface with a nanometer-thick layer of protein containing a bisphosphonate drug. Animal studies indicate that the bone surrounding the implant becomes denser and stronger, ensuring a more durable implant-tissue interface.

References

1. Wynbrandt, J. (2000). *The Excruciating History of Dentistry*. New York: St. Martin's Griffin.
2. Woodforde, J. (1968). *The Strange Story of False Teeth*. London: Routledge & Kegan Paul.
3. James, P. and Thorpe, N. (2015). *Ancient Inventions*. New York: Ballantine Books.
4. Abraham, C.M. (2014). A brief historical perspective on dental implants, their surface coatings and treatments. *Open Dent. J.* 8: 50–55.
5. Wolff, M.S., Allen, K., and Kaim, J. (2007). A 100-year journey from GV Black to minimal surgical intervention. *Compend. Contin. Educ. Dent.* 28 (3): 130–134.
6. Jain, S. and Jain, H. (2017). Legendary Hero: Dr. G.V. Black (1836–1915). *Clin. Diagn. Res.* 11 (5): ZB01–ZB04.
7. Allen, C. (1685). *The Operator for the Teeth*. John White: York.
8. Obwegeser, H.L. (1959). Experiences with subperiosteal implants. *Oral Surg. Oral Med. Oral Pathol.* 12 (7): 777–786.
9. Schou, S., Pallesen, L., Hjørting-Hansen, E. et al. (2000). A 41-year history of a mandibular subperiosteal implant. *Clin. Oral Implants Res.* 11 (2): 171–178.
10. Orlay, H. (1960). Endodontic splinting treatment in periodontal disease. *Br. Dent. J.* 108: 118–121.
11. Gutmann, J.L. and Levermann, V.M. (2013). Endodontic endosseous implants (diodontic or through the tooth implants). *ENDO (Lond. Engl.)* 7 (4): 299–304.
12. von Fraunhofer, J.A. (1975). Oral implants. In: *Scientific Aspects of Dental Materials* (ed. J.A. von Fraunhofer). London: Butterworths.
13. Linkow, L.I. (1970). Endosseous blade-vent implants: a two-year report. *J. Prosth. Dent.* 23 (4): 441–448.
14. Linkow, L.I., Weiss, C.M. and Weiss, L.B. et al. (1973). Oral Implant, USP 3,729,825. 1 May 1973.
15. Pasqualini, M.E., Tramonte, S.U., and Linkow, L.I. (2016). Half a century of function a retrospective analysis of Tramonte endosteal screw dental implants that lasted 50 and 36 years. A case report. *J. Dental Oral Health* 2 (7): 051–058.
16. Moberg, L.E., Sagulin, G.-B., Per-Åke Köndell, P.-A. et al. (2001). Brånemark System® and ITI Dental Implant System® for treatment of mandibular edentulism. A comparative randomized study: 3-year follow-up. *Clin. Oral Implants Res.* 12: 450–461.
17. Maló, P., Rangert, B., and Nobre, M. (2003). Implants for completely edentulous mandibles: a retrospective clinical study. *Clin. Implant Dent. Relat. Res.* 5 (Suppl.1): 2–9.

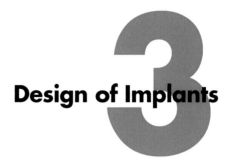

Design of Implants

The modern endosseous dental implant was invented by the Swedish orthopedic surgeon Per-Ingvar Brånemark in 1969. Brånemark's concept was for a cylindrical surgical fixture to be placed into the jawbone and allowed to fuse with the bone over a few months, replacing the root of a missing tooth. After osseointegration, the root-form implant serves as a substrate to hold a replacement tooth or other prosthesis although it should be mentioned that the original Brånemark system was designed for the edentulous jaw rather than single-tooth replacement [1–3]. Because the dental implant is fused to the jawbone, it is very stable and mimics a natural tooth root in that it, and its associated prosthesis, can be independent of adjacent teeth.

Osseointegration, as discussed in earlier chapters, is governed by many factors such as the patient's bone quality, the presence of infections such as peri-implantitis, the type and magnitude of external loading modes, the implant design, the surgical procedure and even corrosion interactions between implant and the abutment or prosthetic crown. Any of these factors, alone or in combination with others, can increase the failure rate of osseointegration. This, in turn, can lead to the implant being lost owing to unsatisfactory or imperfect osseointegration between bone and implant.

Most dental implants are fabricated from titanium or one of its alloys although, as reviewed in the Chapter 2, many other materials have been evaluated as implant materials in the past. The major advantage of titanium and titanium alloys is that they are virtually chemically inert, have great strength and are biocompatible. It is the latter property that allows them to integrate with bone without being recognized as a foreign object by the body.

Today, most implant-supported prostheses replace single missing teeth or address partially edentulous areas; in the latter situation, the final prosthesis

The ADA Practical Guide to Dental Implants, First Edition. Luigi O. Massa and J. Anthony von Fraunhofer.
© 2021 The American Dental Association. Published 2021 by John Wiley & Sons, Inc.

resembles a fixed bridge (see Chapter 4). There is also a growing use of implants for full arch prostheses, either fixed or removable.

The Endosseous Implant

The basic design of an endosseous implant, abutment, and prosthetic crown is shown in Fig. 3.1 and the intended function of the dental implant is shown in Fig. 3.2.

The body of the implant, also known as the *fixture*, is the component that is inserted into bone where it osseointegrates. The upper (coronal) end of the fixture is the collar or crest module, and this is surmounted by the platform or abutment interface.

The Implant Body and Surface

The function of the osseointegrated endosseous implant is to transfer occlusal and masticatory forces from the prosthesis to its surrounding biological tissues. Thus, its primary functional objective is to manage biomechanical loads by dissipating and distributing the applied forces such that the functions of the implant-supported prosthesis are optimized.

Achieving this objective depends on three factors:

- Successful osseointegration with the surrounding bone.
- The nature, magnitude and directionality of the applied forces.
- The surface area of the implant/bone interface over which the force is distributed.

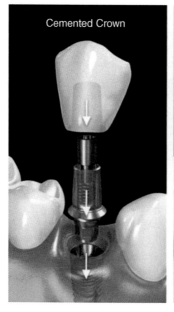
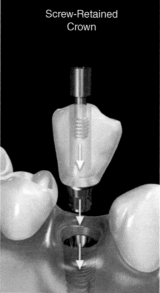

Figure 3.1 The basic implant, abutment, and prosthesis (*Source*: Courtesy of Implant Direct).

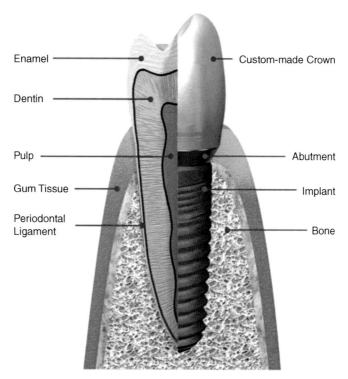

Enamel

Dentin

Pulp

Gum Tissue

Periodontal
Ligament

Custom-made Crown

Abutment

Implant

Bone

Figure 3.2 Comparison of a natural tooth root and an artificial (implant) tooth root (*Source*: Courtesy of Implant Direct).

The cylindrical body of the implant may be smooth, threaded, hollow, or vented. Under compressive (masticatory) loading, a smooth (non-threaded) cylindrical fixture may essentially experience a shear-type force at the implant-bone interface. To alleviate such forces, the fixture surface must be modified to ensure effective and retentive osseointegration. Such surface modifications include providing micro-retention characteristics such as surface roughening, hydroxyapatite (HA) coatings and titanium-plasma spraying. Such micro-retention surface modifications tend to be important for both plane cylindrical fixtures and the more common threaded implants.

Providing the fixture surface with threads came about through further studies by Brånemark and co-workers on osseointegration [4]. This study indicated that the live bone would remodel into the screw shape of an implant, leading to a functional contact for the implant. Consequently, the most common approach to the interfacial stress problem is to provide the implant surface with threading and to taper the implant. It should be noted, however, that although implant fixtures customarily having a threaded, conical shape, they are not "screwed" into the bone but rely upon a retentive fit into a pre-drilled hole or osteotomy cavity.

Many thread designs or shapes are used for dental implants, Fig. 3.3:

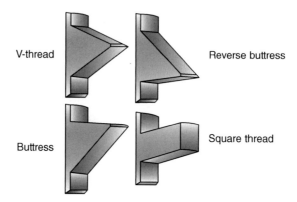

Figure 3.3 Thread designs.

Table 3.1 Purpose of thread designs.

Thread Shape	Designated purpose
Square	Optimal surface area for transmitting compressive load to the bone/ implant interface
Buttress	Optimal for resistance to both pullout (tensile) and/or compressive forces
Reverse buttress	Greater resistance to pullout (tensile) forces
V-shape	Standard (universal) thread pattern

Table 3.2 Thread profiles used by various implant manufacturers.

Thread profile	Manufacturer
Square	Brånemark
V-thread	Brånemark system (Nobel Biocare)
	Screw-vent (Zimmer Dental)
	Certain (Biomet 3)
Buttress	Inclusive tapered implant (Glidewell Laboratories)
	Straumann Standard (Straumann USA)
Reverse buttress	NobelReplace (Nobel Biocare)

Each shape has certain advantages and/or designated purpose, Table 3.1, and each manufacturer has their preferred thread profile, several which are shown in Table 3.2. The V-shape thread, however, is not common with oral implants.

Manufacturers often indicate the characteristics of the threads used on their fixtures, Fig. 3.4. The pitch of a thread is the number of threads per inch (TPI) applied to a single diameter cylinder; a fine-pitch screw has more TPI than a coarse pitch thread. The angle of the thread indicates the steepness of the screw thread (i.e., the "sharpness") whereas the depth indicated is the height of the individual thread above the shank of the screw. Sharper threads have smaller angles and greater thread angles that tend to facilitate bone expansion for greater implant stability. Greater thread depths and coarser thread fixtures are often used to ensure better osseointegration with a dense bony socket.

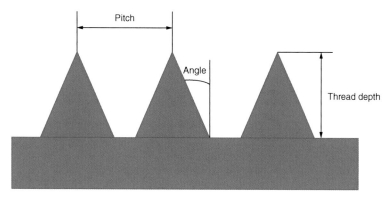

Figure 3.4 Thread characteristics.

It should be mentioned that some implants do incorporate "self-tapping" screw threads but it is not clear at this stage whether this approach improves bony apposition and osseointegration. However, a self-tapping grooved design of the fixture can simplify the surgical protocol. Further, using self-tapping fixtures does reduce the risk of burning or other damage during preparation of the bone during cavity preparation. This may be particularly true with osteotomies for longer implants when providing adequate and effective irrigation deep within the osteotomy during the surgical procedure can be less predictable.

Some manufacturers also fabricate implants with vertical grooves and transecting holes or apertures as additional methods of improving fixture stabilization. The presence of grooving and/or vents permits bony ingrowth which, in turn, prevents rotation of the fixture.

As mentioned earlier, another advance in implant design and fabrication is modification of the implant surface to improve osseointegration and stability, as well as enhance the durability of the integration. Clinical research indicates that roughened surfaces appear to achieve superior osseointegration than smoother, machined surfaces and provide better resistance to torque removal. On the other hand, there are indications that the implants with the roughest surfaces near the coronal aspect may harbor bacteria, leading to chronic implant failure due to bacterially-related peri-implantitis.

The more recent literature suggests that acid-etched surfaces may currently have the optimal degree of surface roughness. This improved osseointegration has been ascribed to the acid-etched surfaces providing increased real surface area and greater surface contour for bone contact and integration. Interestingly, it appears that acid-etched and smooth surfaces are less conducive to bacterial colonization and contamination [5].

Further, some manufacturers coat implant surfaces with HA to encourage new bone growth. In theory, such surface coatings should enhance osseointegration because they provide a more wettable surface and closer osteocyte apposition. HA coatings are also thought to accelerate initial osseointegration which should improve post-surgical stabilization of implants with such surface treatments when placed in less dense bone. A meta-analysis of the survival of HA-coated implants indicates that the survival rates reported for HA-coated implants were similar to the survival rates reported for uncoated titanium implants.

Resorption (or breakdown) of the HA coating did not compromise the long-term survival of dental implants [6]. Finally, most implants have a rounded apical area to facilitate vertical sinus augmentation.

Mini Dental Implants

Another innovation in implant design is the mini-dental implant. The quantity and quality of the remaining bone play a major role in determining whether it is possible to place regular diameter implants which typically have a minimum 3 mm platform. However, in situations where the alveolar ridge is less than 4 mm in width, using a regular width fixture is contra-indicated because of the increased risk of implant exposure. Another situation in which a regular-diameter implant might be considered but is contra-indicated is when there is a restricted space between the roots of the teeth. In such cases, there is an increased risk of periodontal ligament damage of adjacent teeth.

It is possible to address such width constraints on fixtures by increasing bone volume through grafts, osteogenic distraction, or orthodontics. Such procedures may be effective; however, they may not only increase the costs for patients but also carry such risks as unpredictable bone resorption, the possibility of regenerative membrane exposure and prolonged treatment times in situations where the space is restricted. Understandably, some patients decline to undergo such procedures, and this is where mini-implants become a viable treatment option.

Narrow-diameter, as well as shorter length implants, are a good treatment option for sites with suboptimal bone. Such areas of limited bone width typically include severely resorbed mandibular ridges and the central/lateral incisors with their narrow mesio-distal space. Consequently, many studies have reported the use of narrow implants to solve non-ideal clinical situations [7], either alone or in combination with a variety of surgical techniques such as allografts or through guided surgery. Narrow implants appear to be a valid solution in treating localized narrow bony defects in the anterior area with reduced spaces between the natural teeth [8]. Likewise, when the edentulous maxilla is affected by bone resorption, it is difficult to place standard diameter implants. In such situations, narrow diameter titanium-zirconium (Ti-Zr) alloy implants have been proposed for the support of maxillary overdentures and the superior mechanical properties of Ti-Zr compared to Ti is a significant advantage [9].

Despite their undoubted clinical advantages for certain situations, there are indications that the clinical use of narrow diameter implants should be limited to low stress areas, i.e., those subjected to lower masticatory loading.

The Implant Cervical Portion

The crest module of an endosseous implant is the coronal portion of the fixture that retains the prosthetic component. As such, it is the transition zone between the fixture body and the trans-osteal region of the implant at the ridge crest, comprising the implant collar and implant abutment interface. The collar is customarily smooth and increases in diameter from the abutment interface downwards to the fixture body. This cervical slope is designed to prevent or at least reduce gingival recession. Should implant exposure occur, then the cervical slope will enable the margin location to be modified for improved esthetics.

The cervical portion of the implant has shown significant evolution over the years. With the original endosseous root implants, the entire fixture was machined out of titanium or one of its alloys. With the advent of surface texturing, it was assumed that the cervical portion of the implant should also be a machined and textured collar to allow for the periodontal tissues to adapt to it. In most cases, however, bone was found to draw back to the area of the rough-smooth junction.

More recently, there is now greater appreciation of the need to optimize bone retention when the cervical portion of the implant is textured like the rest of the implant body. With many implant designs, the region between the collar and the fixture body may have micro-threads or circular grooves. These features may improve osseointegration close to the collar by increasing overall bone-implant contact and, in turn, improving the system's resistance to oblique forces acting on the prosthesis and implant.

The Abutment Connection

The abutment is the portion of the fixture that both supports and retains the prosthesis or implant superstructure. Abutments fall into three broad categories:

- Screw retention
- Cement retention
- Attachments

and these abutments may be straight or angled, depending on the final prosthesis or superstructure.

It should be stated, however, that dental implant systems can be divided into two types, known as *one-step* and *two-step implant systems*. The one-step system has a single-unit design in which the implant is integrated with the abutment.

Although there are some advantages to having a single integrated system, such as permitting immediate restoration of the edentulous area. But the major disadvantage of the one-piece implant system is that it can cause failure because the abutment is exposed and is superior to the gingival area. One consequence of this is that the abutment is subjected to early loading before osseointegration has been achieved.

In contrast, with the two-piece implant system, the fixture and the abutment are separate entities. During the surgical (osteotomy) procedure, the fixture can be completely buried in the bone during bone healing. Consequently, the fixture may be shielded or protected from early loading and this results in higher potential for uncomplicated bone healing and osseointegration. Nevertheless, despite the more predictable osseointegration with the two-piece implant system, some complications can arise. Because the abutment and fixture of the two-piece implant system are independent, the abutment has to be anchored to the fixture by an abutment central screw. This anchorage is obviously important when the implant system is loaded.

In particular, under loading, the abutment central screw and the abutment itself can be subjected to high stresses, which can lead to loosening of the central screw and abutment. It is also possible for micro-gaps to develop between the abutment and fixture due to sliding and deformation of both components when the system is under loading. Any micro-gaps at the fixture–abutment interface can increase bacterial concentrations in this region and act as a nexus for infection.

Clearly, in order to eliminate or at least reduce possible adverse effects arising from any "looseness" at the junction area of the implant to the abutment, an anti-rotational, indexing configuration is most ideal, especially for single tooth implants. In early implants, this requirement was satisfied through an external hexagonal configuration, but the current preference of implant manufacturers is for internal connections.

This approach has three main advantages, namely greater stability, a decreased incidence of loosening screws and fixture maintenance is greatly simplified. Further, the internal connection, which is routinely deeper than the external hex, ensures a greater depth of interlocking for the segments combined with more certain indexing and better retention. However, because the central screw limits abutment displacement, it can still fracture under loading and even abutment fracture can occur with increased implant diameters. The reason for this occurring is that the implant diameter affects the maximum stress on different parts of the implant system under different contact conditions. For this reason, most manufacturers have adopted *unidiameter* abutments. This simplifies the surgical process and reduces surgical time, allowing assembly of implants with different diameter sizes, Nevertheless, the central screw can still loosen, undergo plastic deformation and fracture. In fact, it is known that fracture of the dental implant and the abutment also can occur due to the internal connection. Whether this occurs depends upon the loading conditions despite the bone and implant being satisfactorily osseointegrated.

As a means of overcoming possible complications with the two-piece implant system such as potential microleakage, some implant companies have adopted the Morse taper design for the interface between the implant and abutment. The Morse taper[1] design uses internal hexagons and octagons on the abutment and implant, respectively. This design can increase the friction between components because of cold-welding[2] and the interference-fit effect. Nowadays, it is common for implant manufacturers to use both Morse tapers and screw retention to improve locking of the abutment to the fixture.

Overall, the net result is greater stability and the attempt to minimize micro-gap formation at the implant–abutment interface. However, whereas a conical connection with a Morse taper can attempt to prevent central screw fracture by limiting abutment displacement under loading, it appears that the unidiameter abutment can cause abutment fracture with an increase in implant diameter together with screw loosening due to plastic deformation. Should fracture occur within the dental implant system, it is a serious problem because fracture of the abutment and/or central screw not only causes damage to the abutment but can also deform the fixture. Either situation may make it difficult to remove the fractured part from the implant system and possibly damage the fixture during removal of the broken abutment or screw.

A final consideration is that the presence of contaminations such as salivary fluids and blood during treatment as well as surface coatings will change the coefficients of friction between mating surfaces within the implant complex. This, in turn, can affect resistance to screw loosening through the effect of friction on the preload, residual torque and removal torque following assembly of the implant system in the mouth.

Although the amount of removal torque required to loosen the abutment screw is less than the insertion torque, any decrease in the coefficient of friction increases the residual torque and the preload. But, on the other hand, the torsional relaxation and the removal torque will be decreased. The net result is that if the coefficient of friction is decreased, there will be enhanced resistance to screw loosening due to increased residual torque. This suggests that dentists should treat the abutment screw with suitable biocompatible lubricants when assembling the implant system in the mouth. However, in order to reduce the risk of corrosion by contaminants, it might be advisable to use gold-coated screws rather than non-coated screws.

Final Thoughts

The continuing growth and widening variety of implant-supported restorations has stimulated continued development of new implant designs and diverse abutment connections compared to the basic Brånemark design. Consequently, increased versatility and flexibility are a priority for the present (and future) generation of dental implants. One result of this trend is that the single-use of an integrated implant is often contra-indicated because one-piece implants have limited application. In contrast, submergible two-piece implants are much more versatile and adaptable because the abutments can be changed as the application changes.

Another factor is that the choice of implant must fit the current use and any future use that may emerge as a patient's needs or requirements change as other factors affect the dentition. This is particularly true for younger patients because although implants may have long-term service over decades of the patient's life, the clinical demands on the implant may change as the patient ages. Thus, for example, it may be advantageous if the abutment on an implant can be changed at a later date so that the attachment to the implant, i.e., the type of prosthesis, can in turn be changed. Such flexibility is not possible with the integrated single-use implant, but it is achievable with two-piece implants. Clearly, removing a well-osseointegrated unsatisfactory or under-performing fixture would present significant problems for the dentist and should be avoided if at all possible.

Notes

1. The Morse Taper, invented in 1864 by Stephen A. Morse, is a method of joining two rotating machine components. The underlying principle is that of a cone locked into a cone. The trunnion or the male portion and the bore (the female portion) are both uniformly tapered. When the bore is tapped onto the trunnion, they come into intimate contact and the conical taper of the trunnion compresses the walls in the bore as it

expands. The stresses generated inside the materials keep both components fixed together. The Morse taper is also commonly used in orthopedic implants.

2. Cold-welding is a bonding process in which two solids are forced together under high pressure to form a single piece but without the need for the application of external heat.

References

1. Brånemark, P.I., Adell, R., Breine, U. et al. (1969). Intra-osseous anchorage of dental prostheses: I. Experimental studies. *Scand. J. Plast. Reconstr. Surg.* 3: 81–100.
2. Moberg, L.E., Sagulin, G.-B., Per-Åke Köndell, P.-A. et al. (2001). Brånemark System® and ITI Dental Implant System® for treatment of mandibular edentulism. A comparative randomized study: 3-year follow-up. *Clin. Oral Implants Res.* 12: 450–461.
3. Maló, P., Rangert, B., and Nobre, M. (2003). Implants for completely edentulous mandibles: a retrospective clinical study. *Clin. Implant Dent. Relat. Res.* 5 (Suppl.1): 2–9.
4. Albrektsson, T., Brånemark, P.I., Hansson, H.A., and Lindström, J. (1981). Osseointegrated titanium implants. Requirements for ensuring a long-lasting, direct bone-to-implant anchorage in man. *Acta Orthop. Scand.* 52: 155–170.
5. Quirynen, M., De Soete, M., and van Steenberghe, D. (2002). Infectious risks for oral implants: a review of the literature. *Clin. Oral Implants Res.* 13: 1–19.
6. Lee, J.J., Rouhfar, L., and Beirne, O.R. (2000). Survival of hydroxyapatite-coated implants: a meta-analytic review. *J. Oral Maxillofac. Surg.* 58 (12): 1372–1379.
7. André, A., Moustapha, S., Marwan, D. et al. (2015). Use of narrow-diameter implants in the posterior jaw: a systematic review. *Implant Dent.* 24 (3): 294–306.
8. Maiorana, C., King, P., Quaas, S. et al. (2015). Clinical and radiographic evaluation of early loaded narrow-diameter implants: 3 years follow-up. *Clin. Oral Implants Res.* 26: 77–82.
9. Cordaro, L., Torsello, F., di Torresanto, V. et al. (2013). Rehabilitation of an edentulous atrophic maxilla with four unsplinted narrow diameter titanium-zirconium implants supporting an overdenture. *Quintessence Int.* 44 (1): 37–43.

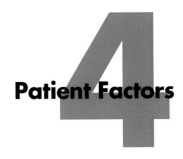

Patient Factors

A basic principle taught in dental school is that both systemic health and oral health are important factors that must be considered when any surgical procedure is performed. This principle covers almost all dental procedures because extractions, cavity preparations, gingivectomies, scaling and polishing, root planing and deep periodontal probing are invasive and surgical in nature. Obviously, site preparation and placing dental implants must be considered to be surgical procedures.

Systemic and Oral Health and Implants

Many systemic conditions have traditionally been considered to be important factors in the success, or failure, of dental implants, Table 4.1; the conditions are listed in alphabetical order.

Clinical studies suggest, however, that most systemic disease or conditions do not significantly increase the risk for implant failure to integrate. There are, however, exceptions to this general rule. Dental implant failure is a possibility for patients diagnosed with RA and diabetes, both of which cause the body to heal at a slower pace and have a higher risk of infection, as well as potentially compromising osseointegration.

The use of certain medications can also lead to dental implant failure, notably through poor osseointegration [1]. Recent research studies indicate that proton pump inhibitors (PPIs), commonly used for the treatment of gastric-acid related disorders, may affect bone regeneration and the osseointegration process, causing an increased risk of deterioration of bone metabolism and impaired bone healing [2]. Likewise, it has been reported that patients using selective serotonin

The ADA Practical Guide to Dental Implants, First Edition. Luigi O. Massa and J. Anthony von Fraunhofer.
© 2021 The American Dental Association. Published 2021 by John Wiley & Sons, Inc.

Table 4.1 Systemic health conditions considered to adversely impact dental implants.

Chemotherapy
Diabetes
Hemophilia
Immunological disorders
Lupus and lichen planus
Malabsorption syndromes
Osteoporosis and osteopenia
Paget's disease
Polycythemia vera
Prolonged bisphosphonate treatment
Radiation treatment of head and neck cancer
Rheumatoid arthritis (RA)
Sjögren's syndrome
Uncontrolled diabetes
Uncontrolled hypertension

reuptake inhibitors (SSRIs) were found to be three times more likely to experience early implant failure than nonusers [3]. Although the findings did not reach statistical significance, they did suggest that SSRIs may lead to an increase in the rate of osseointegration failure.

Although the consensus is that systemic diseases should not be a problem regarding patient selection for implants, there is some evidence that the presence of diabetes mellitus does adversely affect dental implant outcomes [4]. Consequently, dentists should advise patients with medical issues to consult their physicians before undergoing any dental surgery procedure and, when in doubt, the dentist should personally consult with that physician prior to performing any surgical procedure. This is particularly true for patients on blood thinners and those suffering from hypertension.

Patients with the blood disorders, hemophilia[1] and polycythemia vera[2] as well as patients with heart conditions or those who have received arterial stents should always be of concern regarding implants. In the case of patients with polycythemia vera (i.e., a hematocrit >45 for males and >42 for females), anticlotting (anti-platelet) medications such as hydroxyurea (Hydrea®), aspirin and dipyridamole (Persantine®) are often prescribed. Blood thinners are commonly prescribed for patients with heart conditions and to prevent strokes and heart attacks as well as to treat and prevent blood clots; these medications include aspirin, chlopidogrel (Plavix®), apixaban (Eliquis®), warfarin (Coumadin®), rivaroxaban (Xarelto®), and dabigatran (Pradaxa®). Patients who have received stents are also placed on blood thinners for a short period. With patients experiencing any of these conditions or taking such medications, caution must be exercised before undertaking any surgical procedure, including site preparation for implant placement.

At first glance, the caution regarding the potential effects of bisphosphonate therapy on the success of dental implants might appear to be obvious. Bisphosphonates are pharmaceuticals that slow down or prevent bone loss and are recommended for strengthening bones. They are the treatment of choice for osteoporosis and Paget's disease as well as a method of treating hypercalcemia and hyperkalemia, i.e., elevated calcium and potassium levels such as those in certain cancer patients. The therapeutic action of bisphosphonates is through inhibiting osteoclastic activity and promoting more effective osteoblastic activity. Although the optimal duration of bisphosphonate treatment is not known, apparently most benefits occur within the first five years of therapy. Long-term bisphosphonate treatment, however, is reported to lead to atypical femur fractures and osteonecrosis of the jaw as well as esophageal cancer. Consequently, bisphosphonate treatment is customarily reviewed every three to five years and dentists should be cautious when considering dental implants for patients receiving bisphosphonates.

Oral health factors and conditions that may impact the success of dental implants are indicated in Table 4.2. We consider the primary predictors of implant failure are unresolved caries or infection, certain systemic diseases, smoking, advanced age, chronic periodontitis and poor bone quality. Of these oral health factors, the most important appear to be infection and bone quality.

Table 4.2   Oral health factors in implant success or failure.

Bone quality and availability at the implant site
Periodontal disease
Infection
Rampant dental caries
Implant placement adjacent to an existing lesion, e.g., a cyst
Immediate implant placement if extraction necessitated by infection or periodontal disease
Poor oral hygiene
Patient age and gender
Systemic or jaw osteoporosis

However, as is discussed in later chapters, clinical predictors of implant success or failure can include implant location, short implants, acentric loading, an inadequate number of implants, parafunctional habits and absence/loss of implant integration with hard and soft tissues. Inappropriate prosthesis design also may contribute to implant failure.

Infection

Any oral infection is likely to cause problems with dental implants but the conditions that are of the greatest concern are indicated in Table 4.3.

Table 4.3   Oral infections hazardous to dental implants.

Pathology at or in close proximity to the implant site
Infected tooth sockets
Acute or chronic periodontitis
Placement adjacent to an undiagnosed endodontically-involved tooth

Clinicians must be vigilant regarding bacterial infections, notably apical lesions, periodontal disease and dental caries, all of which have to be addressed before undertaking any implant procedure. Although implant failure or impaired osseointegration is not inevitable, the prognosis may be compromised when it is placed adjacent to an existing lesion, e.g., a cyst, or when rampant caries or periodontal (chronic or acute) disease exists in adjacent teeth. Thus, for example, although the incidence of peri-mucositis is reported to be >50% and that of peri-implantitis >12%, the rate of confirmed implant infection is stated to be ≤2.1% [5]. Likewise, provided there has been appropriate antimicrobial treatment, bone loss is not too severe and there is adequate oral hygiene, dental implants can remain functional when there has been infection or periodontal disease [6].

Clinical studies indicate that the administration of prophylactic antibiotics significantly reduces the prevalence of dental implant failure under ordinary conditions [7]. Further, no differences were found in dental implant failures and infections between patients prescribed preoperative antibiotics and those received both preoperative and postoperative antibiotics. However, other work suggests that antibiotic therapy may have no effect on early implant failure.

Poor oral hygiene is also an important warning sign for the clinician since gingivitis and periodontal disease can easily recur after implant placement unless patients are meticulous regarding regular brushing and flossing. Osseointegration following placement of an implant can be impaired due to adverse periodontal conditions.

It is also worth mentioning that there appears to be a greater prevalence of oral candidiasis (oral thrush) in recent years. Although *Candida albicans* is normally present in the oral cavity, it appears that overgrowth and proliferation is becoming more common in the general population in addition to traditionally being most common in babies, older adults and patients with impaired immune systems. Anecdotal reports suggest that one cause possibly contributing to the increased occurrence of oral candidiasis is the greater use of peroxide-containing dentifrices and in-home tooth bleaching systems. Research studies, however, indicate that these tooth bleaching agents have antimicrobial properties [8] and many are cytotoxic [9]. It should also be noted that it is uncertain whether candidiasis will adversely affect implants although colonization is clearly a possibility.

Bone Quality

There are numerous risk factors for dental implant failure [10], these include poor bone quality, chronic periodontitis, certain systemic diseases, smoking, and unresolved caries or infection. As will be discussed in later chapters, clinical predictors of implant success or failure include implant location, short implants, acentric loading, an inadequate number of implants, parafunctional habits and absence/loss of implant integration with hard and soft tissues. Inappropriate prosthetic design also may contribute to implant failure. Nevertheless, after infection, bone quality appears to be the most important factor in implant success and failure.

Bone quality may be categorized as being one of four types, Table 4.4.

The potential success of an implant is determined, often in large part, by the quality of bone into which it is to be inserted, Fig. 4.1.

Ideally, the patient should have Type I or Type II bone if the highest rate of success is to be achieved. Patients with Type III or IV bone are less likely to be good candidates for dental implants, as noted in Table 4.2 and Fig. 4.1. Obviously, patients suffering from osteoporosis present a greater risk for implant failure.

Table 4.4 Type of bone.

Bone Type	Characteristics
Type I	Entire jaw comprises homogenous compact bone
Type II	Core of dense trabecular bone surrounded by thick layer of compact bone
Type III	Thin layer of cortical bone surrounding core of dense trabecular bone
Type IV	Core of low density trabecular bone surrounded by thin layer of cortical bone

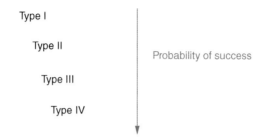

Figure 4.1 Effect of bone type on implant success.

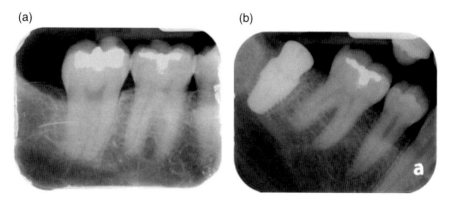

Figure 4.2 (a) Tooth #31 requiring extraction due to vertical crack transecting the tooth. (b). Immediate implant placement following extraction of tooth #31 shown in (a).

Immediate implant placement is justified following tooth extraction because of trauma or tooth cracking provided that there is good or satisfactory bone quality and quantity at the extraction site, Fig. 4.2a,b. Under these circumstances, placing an immediate implant should be straightforward.

Evaluation and determination of bone quality are both discussed in later chapters, together with the need for such considerations when placing implants into post-extraction healed bone and for immediate implant (fresh extraction) sites.

Clinical studies indicate that many patient factors such as age, gender, body mass index (BMI) or, indeed, the implant site and even smoking should have little significant impact on implant survival. It should be noted, however, that the condition of the jawbone is both age- and site-specific although increased age apparently does not affect the clinical potential for osseointegration. Further, the rate of crestal bone resorption occurring around oral implants is, apparently, not affected or determined by patient age. On the other hand, the jaw site is related to osseointegration potential with such integration tending to be more successful with mandibular sites than maxillary sites.

This difference in osseointegration potential possibly could be that jawbone quality and quantity is more commonly compromised in maxillary than in mandibular sites. However, clinical reports suggest that high rates of implant success are achievable in maxillary sites, even those with low trabecular bone density, if an adequate volume of bone exists to accommodate the implants. In addition to numerous other factors already mentioned, these observations were based on short-term evidence and may be questionable in the long-term.

Although the rate of crestal bone resorption around oral implants is usually low and may not be site-specific, there is some evidence that implants, placed at the crestal level, showed greater peri-implant bone stability during the 1-year follow-up [11]. Although the rate of crestal bone resorption around oral implants is usually low and may not be site-specific, it may be greater in sites with less preoperative resorption associated with shorter periods of edentulism [12] and potentially could jeopardize long-term implant outcomes. Accordingly, we feel that even for tooth extractions unrelated to caries, periodontal disease or endodontic infection, healing for at least six months should be encouraged following extraction to ensure stable resorption and bone consolidation at the implant site.

If the bone profile at the proposed implant site is disadvantageous, recreating tissue profile is extremely challenging especially if time has elapsed from tooth loss. Accordingly, as discussed later under surgical procedures, maintaining the correct bone profile is important during site preparation.

Patient Factors

Patient attitude and expectations of implants often have a significant impact on the success of implants. Many patients are displeased and often disappointed to learn that there might be an extended period between implant placement and fabrication of a restoration. Whether mental attitudes can affect implant success is unknown but delays and impatience probably do not contribute to osseointegration. Clearly, the clinician needs to apprise the patient of all aspects of placing implants so that the patient understands what the procedure involves before treatment is initiated.

Clinical studies indicate that many patient factors such as age, gender, BMI or, indeed, the implant site and even smoking should have little significant impact on implant survival. Thus, the overall success rate of oral implants is claimed to be about 95% and appears to be almost independent of the patient. This statement is misleading, if not inaccurate. Osteoporosis, uncontrolled hypertension and possibly diabetes mellitus all present risks to implant success as do certain medications, e.g., bisphosphonates. Post-placement patient factors such as poor oral hygiene, gingivitis, plaque, and calculus accretion around the implant will encourage gingival recession around the implant. With continued accumulation of plaque and calculus around the implant/gingival margin, pockets will deepen, leading to bone loss. As the latter progresses, the stability of the implant will steadily decrease and might potentially lead to failure.

Likewise, chewing on pipe stems, pens and pencils and other parafunctional activities, including bruxism, can overload the implant or cause lateral stresses. Lateral displacements of implants will inevitably result in loosening of the implant, eventually resulting in failure. For this reason, patients subject to bruxism should be encouraged to wear a custom-fitted night guard to avoid undue stress being placed on the implant.

Implants, by definition, have no periodontal ligament and thus no proprioception. Consequently, normal reactions by the dentate patient when biting down on very hard objects cannot occur with restorations placed on implants. As a result, heavy masticatory loads may result in failure of restorations and, worse, fracture of parts of the implant complex. Without proprioception, such failure of restorations and/or implants may be undetected by the patient, potentially leading to further and potentially catastrophic failures. For this reason, implant patients must be encouraged to have routine (at least six month) follow-ups and dental hygiene appointments to avoid accumulation of plaque and calculus around their implants.

It should be noted, as discussed in later chapters, the factors that do affect implant survival are often those related to the implant itself, notably length and type (cylindrical or tapered) and the surgical technique followed during placement. Evaluation of the potential implant site is discussed in Chapter 7.

Conclusion

Obtaining a thorough and current medical history is imperative to evaluate potential risk factors which can hinder the osseointegration process. The practitioner must also discuss habits that affect success rates such as tobacco use as well as take note of the medications taken by the patient. Lastly, one must perform a complete clinical examination to evaluate factors such as periodontal disease, bruxism, and oral hygiene. While many of the negative factors are not absolute contra-indications to placing an implant, they will guide the practitioner to understand and share the relative risk of the procedure with the patient.

Notes

1. Hemophilia is a blood defect occurring almost exclusively in males which is characterized by delayed clotting of the blood with prolonged or excessive internal or external bleeding after injury or surgery.
2. Polycythemia vera is an uncommon neoplasm causing the bone marrow to make too many red blood cells and which may also result in the overproduction of white blood cells and platelets.

References

1. Ouanounou, A., Hassanpour, S., and Glogauer, M. (2016). The influence of systemic medications on osseointegration of dental implants. *J. Can. Dent. Assoc.* 82 (g7): 1–8.

2. Mester, A., Apostu, D., Ciobanu, L. et al. (2019). The impact of proton pump inhibitors on bone regeneration and implant osseointegration. *Drug Metab. Rev.* 51 (3): 330–339.

3. Altay, M.A. and Sindel, A. (2018). Does the intake of selective serotonin reuptake inhibitors negatively affect dental implant osseointegration? A retrospective study. *J. Oral Implantol.* 44 (4): 260–265.

4. Michaeli, E., Weinberg, I., and Nahlieli, O. (2009). Dental implants in the diabetic patient: systemic and rehabilitative considerations. *Quintessence Int.* 40 (8): 639–645.

5. Powell, C.A., Mealey, B.L., Deas, D.E. et al. (2005). Post-surgical infections: prevalence associated with various periodontal surgical procedures. *J. Periodontol.* 76 (3): 329–333.

6. Blus, C., Szmukler-Moncler, S., Khoury, P. et al. (2015). Immediate implants placed in infected and noninfected sites after atraumatic tooth extraction and placement with ultrasonic bone surgery. *Clin. Implant Dent. Relat. Res.* 17 (Suppl 1): e287–e297.

7. Arduino, P.G., Tirone, F., Schlorin, E. et al. (2015). Single preoperative dose of prophylactic amoxicillin versus a 2-day postoperative course in dental implant surgery: a two-center randomised controlled trial. *Eur. J. Oral Implantol.* 8 (2): 143–149.

8. Napimoga, M.H., de Oliveira, R., Reis, A.F. et al. (2007). In vitro antimicrobial activity of peroxide-based bleaching agents. *Quintessence Int.* 38 (6): e329–e333.

9. Chin, S., Tse, S., Lynch, E. et al. (1991). Is home tooth bleaching gel cytotoxic? *J. Esthet. Rest. Dent.* 3 (5): 162–168.

10. Paquette, D.W., Brodala, N., and Williams, R.C. (2006). Risk factors for endosseous dental implant failure. *Dent. Clin. N. Am.* 50 (3): 361–374.

11. Gatti, C., Gatti, F., Silvestri, M. et al. (2018). A prospective multicenter study on radiographic crestal bone changes around dental implants placed at crestal or subcrestal level: one-year findings. *Int. J. Oral Maxillofac. Implants* 33 (4): 913–918.

12. Bryant, S.R. (1998). The effects of age, jaw site, and bone condition on oral implant outcomes. *Int. J. Prosthodont.* 11 (5): 470–490.

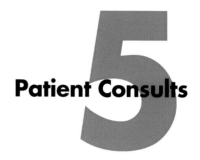

Patient Consults

When consulting with a patient, the modern dental practitioner must inform patients of all the treatment options and arrive at a satisfactory treatment plan. This requires the practitioner to look at the patient in a comprehensive manner so that optimal treatment can be provided.

The successful consultation consists of diagnosing the conditions, educating the patient and understanding the patient's expectations.

Patients will seek the advice of a dentist who performs implants for several reasons, typically those listed in Table 5.1 and reviewed previously in Chapter 1.

However, before addressing the patient's complaints and concerns, the dentist must evaluate the patient.

Evaluating the Patient

There are several important components in the initial patient evaluation. The first is the patient's medical and oral health, as reviewed and discussed in Chapter 4. Provided the patient meets these health criteria, the dentist can initiate a discussion of what treatment the patient wants to have and, in turn, what can be provided. The first thing that the dentist must do in this regard is to inform the patient of their options and let them and their desires lead to the best treatment plan.

The best way to approach this for, say, a complete denture patient, is to outline what those options are along with reasonable expectations of masticatory forces, see Table 5.2.

There are, of course, other factors and these vary with the patient's treatment needs and desires. For example, in a case where the supporting teeth for a

The ADA Practical Guide to Dental Implants, First Edition. Luigi O. Massa and J. Anthony von Fraunhofer.
© 2021 The American Dental Association. Published 2021 by John Wiley & Sons, Inc.

Table 5.1 Patients' complaints.

Loose/ill-fitting dentures
Discomfort
Denture-related halitosis
Mobile/missing teeth
Unattractive smile/teeth
Masticatory pain

Table 5.2 Projected cost and masticatory efficiency of dentures vs implants (Note that costs can vary widely).

The average cost of a complete denture is $1200 but only provides 15% of the dentate bite force.
The cost of an implant overdenture is $7000–$12000 but provides 50% of the dentate bite force.
The cost of fixed implant bridge/bridges is $16000–$20000 but provides 90% of the dentate bite force.

removal partial denture (RPD) are failing or there is a general breakdown of the dentition, replacement with a more stable and satisfactory prosthesis is necessary. However, if the patient has worn RPD's for years and is happy with them, then an overdenture may be an appropriate treatment option. On the other hand, in the situation where a patient has missing teeth that need replacement but is terrified of, or totally averse to, a removable prosthesis, then a fixed implant supported bridge may be the best option.

The bottom line is: the dentist must identify the patient's' needs. In the majority of cases, the latter will fall into one of the following three alternatives:

1. Single-tooth replacement options
2. Partially edentulous options
3. Edentulous options

Treatment Options and the Dentist

Central to the dentist-patient interaction is an appreciation of what implant dentistry can do for the patient, and for the dentist. In restorative dentistry, the crown generally meets three important criteria:

* Long-term success rate
* Predictable outcome
* Low-stress procedure

Surprisingly, implant dentistry meets these same criteria but with the added advantage that the dentist can control the case from start to finish. In many situations, we alone know where we are going in the treatment schema. There are, of course, many other advantages (see Table 5.3), to undertaking dental implant treatment modalities.

Table 5.3 Advantages of implants.

An implant is the single best treatment option in most cases
There is low-stress for the patient
Implant dentistry is the future of dentistry
Implants can satisfy patient demands
Demand for implants is growing because of an aging population and the need for denture
    stabilization
Implants have a 95–97% recorded success rate, higher than any other procedure we
    perform
Implants are the most researched procedure in dentistry
Patient satisfaction is high
Emergency treatment of failing teeth with implants is possible
Immediate temporization is possible in many cases

It should be mentioned that before embarking on devising a treatment plan, the dentist should ensure that the patient is financially viable. Needless to say, the costs involved in constructing diagnostic models, wax ups, CT scans and surgical guides all mount up, even for the simplest cases. If a dental implant or implants are beyond the financial resources of the patient and financing options are not available, then conventional treatment approaches, although less ideal, must be adopted.

The economics and financial aspects of implants were indicated in Table 5.2 and are discussed in much greater detail in Chapter 16.

It is also necessary to assemble or collect data for the treatment plan. Typically, this involves the following:

- Health HX
- Dental HX
- Radiographs
- Cone beam computed tomography (CBCT) if necessary
- Models if necessary

Data collection becomes easier with experience and will allow a quick diagnosis and treatment plan. On the other hand, a quick diagnosis without experience can cause trouble. Likewise, a conservative diagnosis without experience often creates roadblocks to treatment acceptance.

If the requisite data has been collected for the patient and a preliminary treatment plan devised, then constructive interactions become possible. These often involve short presentations showing the patient radiographs and models of their mouths and dentition, and the radiographs and post-op pictures of similar cases that you have performed.

Although the patient-dentist consult can often involve a quasi-sales pitch, this is usually necessary because the patient must agree to certain commitments:

- A significant financial investment.
- Time commitment.
- Complete trust and reliance on the dentist.
- Several visits to the practice for CT scans, radiographs, impressions, etc.
- Some discomfort is possible during the osteotomy.

- A potential delay of weeks or months during osseointegration for edentulous sites.
- The need for temporization if teeth were extracted.

Time spent with the patient will always pay dividends in terms of their satisfaction and your own personal pride in providing expert dental care.

Conclusions

While it is vital to understand how to perform clinical implant procedures, it is equally important to understand how to present the pros and cons to the patient. During the patient consultation, the practitioner must discuss the different treatment modalities as they relate to masticatory forces, cleanability, esthetics, and longevity. Spending time conversing with the patient will help reveal their motivating factors and these will help the practitioner to arrive at a customized treatment plan.

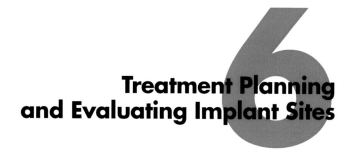

Treatment Planning and Evaluating Implant Sites

Patient desires/perceptions regarding seeking dental implant therapy are based predominantly on the following criteria:

- Function
- Esthetics
- Success rate
- Ability to properly cleanse

Addressing these patient concerns and requirements involves several common scenarios that take advantage of the versatility of dental implants. These are discussed in Chapter 7. However, the first issue that must be addressed by the practitioner is treatment planning. With experience, the average practitioner will undertake this exercise automatically but for the less experienced dentist, Fig. 6.1 indicates the treatment planning steps that should be taken with a new patient.

The first task of the clinician when facing a new patient is a comprehensive systemic and oral health evaluation, as discussed in Chapters 4 and 5. If there are no oral or other (systemic) health issues that could adversely affect the surgical treatment of the patient, then the next task is to determine what the perceived needs and desires of the patient are seeking treatment.

The next issue to be addressed is evaluation of the implant site. The site is evaluated both radiographically and visually. Ideally, both two-dimensional (2D) (traditional radiography) and three-dimensional (3D) cone beam computed tomography (CBCT) are utilized. If CBCT is not available, then "ridge mapping" is a good alternative. Ridge mapping is the process of bone sounding to create a "map" of the bony structure. Both the vertical and the horizontal dimension of bone must be assessed to determine if implant therapy is practical. The basic

The ADA Practical Guide to Dental Implants, First Edition. Luigi O. Massa and J. Anthony von Fraunhofer.
© 2021 The American Dental Association. Published 2021 by John Wiley & Sons, Inc.

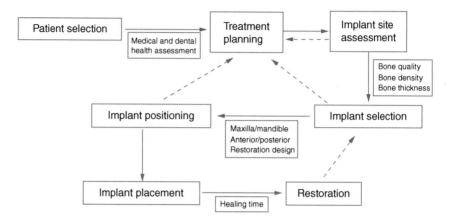

Figure 6.1   Treatment planning for implants.

limitation to implant placement is outlined by "the rule of 6's." This states that there must be 6 mm of vertical and horizontal bone. There must be 6 mm of space from mesial to distal and there must be 6 mm of inter-occlusal space. If these criteria are not met, bone augmentation can be performed.

Bone deficiencies occur for multiple reasons but are primarily due to bone resorption over time following an extraction. It can also occur in the posterior maxilla due to sinus pneumatization. Horizontal deficiency can be corrected with GBR (guided bone regeneration) whereas sinus augmentation can correct vertical deficiency in the posterior maxilla.

Deciding which implant to use is often a matter of personal choice and, as indicated in Chapter 3, there are a plethora of implant systems available to the practitioner. The final decision on implant system selection lies with the dentist but will be impacted by the implant site, the operative conditions and the type of restoration to be placed on the implant(s). Chapter 7 indicates possible implant scenarios which, in turn, will indicate the requirements for the implants to be placed.

The implant selection criteria include those indicated in Table 6.1:

Some of these selection criteria were discussed in Chapter 3 whereas the remainder are addressed here and in subsequent chapters.

Table 6.1   Implant selection criteria.

- Implant design
- Bone level relative to coronal implant position
- Internal connection
- Long-term availability of parts
- Platform switch (horizontal offset)
- Abutments to allow a multitude of restorative choices

If sufficient bone exists, it must be determined whether the implant can be restored properly. Things to consider include the absence or presence of the opposing teeth as well as their condition. Also, the practitioner must consider the angle at which the implant will be placed. Ideally, the implant should be placed along the long axis of the final restoration. If there is excessive off-angle loading, bone loss or restorative failure may occur.

Implant Site Evaluation – Healed Bone

Endosseous implants are used in edentulous areas where there is sufficient healthy bone to accommodate the implant without risk of damage to vital structures. An illustration of a single tooth implant and restoration is shown in Fig. 6.2. Endosseous implants are contra-indicated in situations where there has been excessive ridge resorption. Other contra-indications for endosseous implants include severe malocclusion, bruxism, and parafunctional oral activities such as pipe or pencil chewing.

The practitioner may decide to undertake treatment when certain criteria are satisfied, Table 6.2:

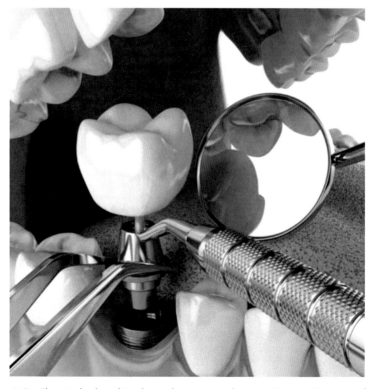

Figure 6.2   The single dental implant, abutment, and crown (Source: Courtesy of Implant Direct).

Table 6.2   Criteria for satisfactory implant placement.

6 mm radiographic height
6 mm of bone width (determined from CBCT or ridge mapping)
6 mm mesial-distal space
6 mm inter-occlusal space
Implant site accessibility

Implant Site Evaluation – Immediate Site

When evaluating a potential extraction/immediate implant placement site, the clinician must evaluate the following:

• Absence of any active infection
• Intact buccal plate
• The likelihood of an atraumatic tooth extraction
• The existence of all walls of bone (Buccal, Lingual/Palatal, Mesial, Distal)
• Sufficient vertical height of bone between the implant site and vital structures
• Insertion torque – of about 25 Ncm

If these criteria are not met, it is best to perform socket preservation and thus delay implant placement.

Although placing a single implant in a healed site is perhaps the simplest and most straightforward of implant procedures, clinicians can run into problems and situations that need to be addressed appropriately to achieve a successful outcome.

Conclusion

The treatment planning discussed in this chapter was largely directed at single/individual implant placement. However, the same rules and criteria apply whether one or several implants are to be placed and regardless of the final restoration. Thus, for example, the rule of 6's should be followed whenever possible. In situations where bone augmentation is deemed necessary, then grafting should be undertaken. In situations where there is restricted space or narrow buccal-lingual bone width at the implant site, then narrow-diameter (mini) implants may be considered.

The following chapter, Chapter 7, indicates the diversity of clinical situations in which implants can be used to address patient problems and requirements. The surgical procedures involved in placing these implants are discussed in Chapters 8–12. The other issue with an implant, namely its restoration, involves deciding on how the prosthetic crown is attached to the abutment, i.e., whether the crown should be screw-retained or cemented in place, and this is discussed in Chapter 13.

Implant Scenarios 7

The versatility and almost universal scope of dental implantology has been stressed throughout this book. Although the average dentist is aware of conventional approaches to addressing the replacement of missing teeth, most may benefit from being apprised of the diversity of options that are now available and which are becoming commonplace in dental implant practices.

The Single Crown

The basic procedure in implant dentistry is the replacement of a missing tooth with a single crown placed on an individual implant, Fig. 7.1 and Fig. 7.2.

The single implant-retained crown replaces a missing tooth and can restore an unattractive or patient-restricted smile, improve masticatory ability and slow down or retard bone loss. When that missing tooth is a central or lateral incisor, implant dentistry obviates previous restorative techniques such as the Maryland bridge and many other procedures. The latter include fixed partial dentures, removable partial dentures (RPDs) and "flippers."

The other major advantage with the single dental implant is that it avoids the need for a three-unit bridge, Fig. 7.3. Since preparing the abutment teeth for the bridge involves loss of sound enamel from the proposed abutment teeth, implant dentistry is clearly a remarkable advance in conserving otherwise sound teeth. This can be an important consideration when the abutment teeth may be compromised by dental caries or periodontal disease.

Another advantage of individually-restored implants compared to bridges is that implants tend to retard continuing bone loss that often occurs at edentulous

---

The ADA Practical Guide to Dental Implants, First Edition. Luigi O. Massa and J. Anthony von Fraunhofer.
© 2021 The American Dental Association. Published 2021 by John Wiley & Sons, Inc.

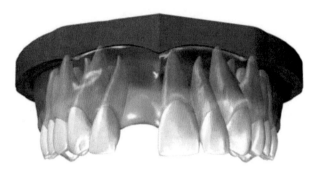

Figure 7.1   The missing tooth syndrome (*Source*: Courtesy of Implant Direct).

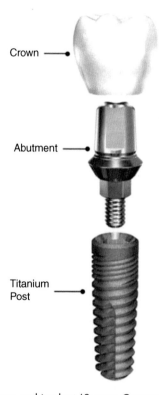

Crown

Abutment

Titanium
Post

Figure 7.2   The single crown and implant (*Source*: Courtesy of Implant Direct).

sites. They can also reduce the risk of dental caries and potential tooth loss because the single implant is considered to be more hygienic than a conventional bridge. However, the need for continued oral hygiene and periodontal maintenance of the implant site must be stressed to avoid the development of pocketing between the implant and its bony and soft-tissue support. This topic is revisited in later chapters.

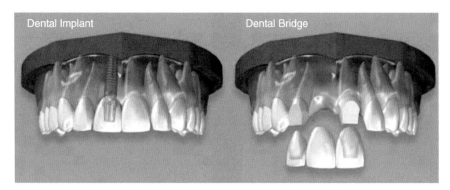

Figure 7.3 The dental implant vs a three-unit bridge (*Source*: Courtesy of Implant Direct).

Implant-Supported Bridgework vs the FPD/RPD

When several teeth are missing, both the dentist and the patient face the difficult task of choosing between a RPD, a fixed partial denture (FPD) or a multi-unit implant bridge. The decision becomes even more difficult and/or problematic when the adjacent teeth are decayed or have periodontal involvement. A further factor in this decision process can be when financial considerations and the overall cost of treatment come into play (see Chapter 17).

As discussed in Chapter 1, most patients do not favor RPDs, especially if they are polymer-based rather than the more expensive but more rigid cast alloy frameworks. FPDs or bridges that span several missing teeth present problems with regard to the stability of the abutment teeth and the potential of overloading the abutment teeth. Recurrent decay of the abutment teeth has the potential to cause premature failure of the restoration. A further consideration can be with the "distal extension area" when there is no distal abutment for the FPD.

Implant bridges allow the practitioner to replace multiple teeth with implant supported prosthetics, Fig. 7.4. It is a generally accepted practice that two implants can restore three to four teeth. This allows for several configurations where one can have a traditional bridge of Retainer/Pontic/Retainer or

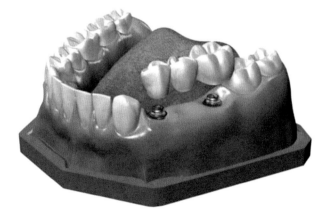

Figure 7.4 Posterior implant bridgework (*Source*: Courtesy of Implant Direct).

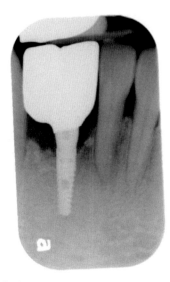

Figure 7.5 Replacing multiple anterior teeth.

Retainer/Pontic/Pontic/Retainer or variations thereof. It is acceptable to have one pontic cantilever either anterior or posterior when the bridge is supported by two implants.

Implants may also be splinted to natural teeth to restore multiple missing teeth, although this restoration should be used with caution. There may be potential complications with the natural tooth because, in contrast to an implant, theoretically the PDL can permit tooth movement such that the implant may differentially take loading to the point of overloading.

Similar considerations apply in the anterior region, Fig. 7.5.

In the authors' opinion, dental implants are the treatment option of choice, and perhaps the standard of care, for the replacement and restoration of multiple missing teeth for both dentate and partially dentate patients.

The Edentulous Patient

As discussed in Chapter 1, treating the edentulous patient is often very challenging for the general dentist. This is especially true when the patient has severely resorbed ridges, flat ridges or, in the case of an upper denture, a shallow palatal vault. In each of these situations, achieving a stable, retentive denture is usually difficult without resorting to retentive aids such as denture fixatives. A further factor with complete dentures is that when they rest on ridges with residual spicules of cancellous bone or following recent extraction(s), the patient can experience severe pain on mastication. Masticatory pain can be ameliorated, at least temporarily, by means of tissue conditioners and resilient liners. However, these measures are temporary and require replacement on a regular basis, which can present problems if the liners are heat-cured and for non-ambulatory patients. Often, the cost and office visits associated with repeated and necessary relining of complete dentures also presents problems.

Other considerations and patient complaints that often impel them to seek implant therapy include those indicated in Table 7.1:

The obvious solution to such problems is the implant over-denture, Fig. 7.6.

The complete denture can be screw-retained (Fig. 7.7a,b). or "snap onto" the implant abutments (Fig. 7.8).

Table 7.1 Patient complaints and dissatisfactions with complete dentures.

Poor denture stability
Lack of retention
Diminished masticatory forces
Pain due to impinging nerve on severely resorbed mandible
Speech impairment
Impaired taste and thermal sensitivity with upper dentures
Oral malodor

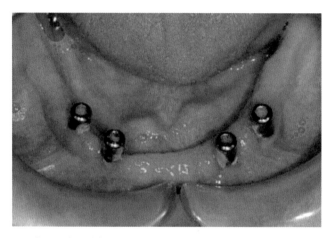

Figure 7.6 Implants placed for an implant-supported over-denture.

(a)   (b)

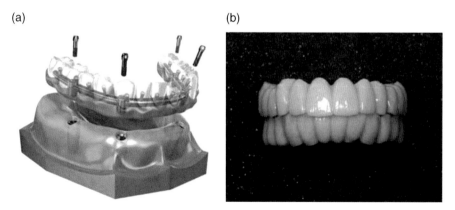

Figure 7.7 (a) Fixed implant-supported bridge (*Source*: Courtesy of Implant Direct). (b) Fixed zirconia implant-supported bridge.

There are two basic choices for the "terminal dentition" or the edentulous patient. The first option is the implant over-denture. The second option is the fixed implant bridge(s).

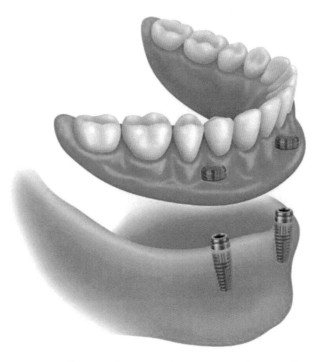

Figure 7.8   Snap-on implant overdenture (*Source*: Courtesy of Zest Anchor).

Implant Over-denture

The implant over-denture is an implant and tissue-supported prosthesis. Generally, two to four implants are placed per arch to stabilize the denture. Specific abutments are placed on the implants and corresponding attachments are processed into the denture to create a "snapping-in" of the denture. The patient should remove the appliance to clean daily. The patient is instructed to not sleep with the appliance. Recommended scheduled maintenance includes implant and prosthesis cleaning at 6-month intervals, replacing denture attachments every six months–one year, and relining the appliance every two to five years. Abutments may need to be replaced after five years due to wear although wear patterns can be variable due to patient factors.

Fixed Implant Bridge(S)

Fixed implant bridges are completely implant-supported screw-retained prosthesis. Generally, four to six implants are used to support the prosthesis. Materials used include milled bars (chrome–cobalt or titanium) and processed acrylic or milled prosthesis (poly-methyl methacrylate) [PMMA] or zirconia). Increasingly, zirconia is becoming the material of choice for these prostheses due to its strength, durability, and biocompatibility. When zirconia is utilized, the prosthesis is fabricated much like the traditional FPD, potentially allowing for better cleansability. Patients are educated in the use of water flosser devices as well as floss threaders.

Regular scheduled maintenance for fixed implant bridges include implant and prosthesis cleaning every six months, appliance removal every one to two years with possible screw replacement.

Regardless of the stabilization/retention method adopted, implant-supported dentures successfully address, if not eliminate, most if not all the patient issues with CDs listed in Table 7.1. With implant-retained dentures, such problems as denture slipping, poor stability, impaired masticatory performance and masticatory pain become things of the past for the edentulous patient [1–3].

Conclusions

Dental implants have clearly had a major impact on restorative dentistry. The versatility of dental implants allows for single-tooth replacement, multiple-tooth replacement, and full-arch tooth replacement. There are numerous benefits of implant treatment in comparison to traditional restorative dentistry. These benefits include reducing unnecessary tooth preparation, creating a more hygienic tooth replacement, increasing denture stabilization, and creating fixed restorative treatments for edentulous patients.

References

1. Fueki, K., Kimoto, K., Ogawa, T. et al. (2007). Effect of implant-supported or retained dentures on masticatory performance: a systematic review. *J. Prosth. Dent.* 98 (6): 470–477.
2. Hyland, R., Ellis, J., Thomason, M. et al. (2009). A qualitative study on patient perspectives of how conventional and implant-supported dentures affect eating. *J. Dent.* 37 (9): 718–723.
3. Zembic, A. and Wismeijer, D. (2014). Patient-reported outcomes of maxillary implant-supported overdentures compared with conventional dentures. *Clin. Oral Implants Res.* 25 (4): 441–450.

Implant Surgery: Simple Healed Sites

The first step in planning implant surgery is to open a dialogue with the patient to identify the problem, as discussed in Chapters 4–6. After discussing costs, outlining the procedures involved and deciding upon the optimum treatment plan, the most important task is to perform a patient evaluation and collect essential data, Table 8.1.

Many dentists do not have ready access to a CBCT (cone beam computed tomography) system and, when weighing whether to embark on implant surgery, they often ask whether CBCT's are necessary. The answer to this question is that *No, they are not essential* and, in fact, millions of implants have been placed without CBCT although there is no doubt that they can be very useful during treatment planning. One alternative to CBCT is bone sounding which, in most cases, can provide sufficient information for clinical decision making. However, as discussed below, it is important for the dentist to have available solid information on the bony parameters of the implant site. In the absence of a CBCT image, it is advisable to reflect a full thickness flap for the first 50 implant placements until the operator gains sufficient experience to readily visualize the bony architecture prior to surgery.

Treatment Agenda

Replacing a missing or extracted single (free-standing) tooth is the most common implant procedure performed. It is the most basic implant procedure in that there is no need for preparation of abutment teeth for a traditional bridge. Even although this procedure is surgical in nature, it is less invasive in that removal of enamel is an irreversible procedure. Bone and soft tissue can be regenerated

The ADA Practical Guide to Dental Implants, First Edition. Luigi O. Massa and J. Anthony von Fraunhofer.
© 2021 The American Dental Association. Published 2021 by John Wiley & Sons, Inc.

Table 8.1   Data collection for treatment planning.

Health history
Dental history
Radiographs
CBCT[a], if necessary
Models, if necessary

[a] CBCT: Cone beam computed tomography (also known as cone beam volume CT, C-arm CT or flat panel CT) is an imaging technique consisting of X-ray computed tomography where the X-rays directed at the subject diverge to form a cone.

Table 8.2   Bone factors in implant planning (≥ denotes greater than or equal to, or simply "no less than").

Radiographic height of available bone (≥6 mm)
CT width, ridge mapping (≥6 mm)
Inter-occlusal space (≥6 mm)
M-D width (≥6 mm)
Bone quality
Accessibility

through grafting procedures. Generally, the long-term prognosis is better for a single implant than for a traditional bridge. Further, although the initial cost may be higher for a single implant, the long-term cost is lower than for a traditional bridge. Also, replacing a single tooth will simplify possible future retention of prostheses such as FPD's, RPD's, and CD's.

Systemic and Dental History

As discussed in Chapter 4, the following conditions are relative contra-indications for implant surgery:

- Uncontrolled hypertension
- Uncontrolled diabetes
- IV bisphosphonates
- Periodontal disease (increases risk of peri-implantitis)
- Smoking

Obviously, absence of active infection is strongly advised. Although smoking may not be a direct contra-indication to implant surgery, advising the patient to avoid smoking for 48 hours post-surgery may help reduce complications [1].

Most clinical factors impacting the decision to perform implant surgery are discussed in detail in Chapters 4–7. Nevertheless, it is useful to repeat them here as Tables 8.2 and 8.3 indicate the implant site considerations and treatment factors that must be decided on before surgery.

Regarding bone quality and the bony parameters surrounding the implant site, having a CBCT scan available does simplify matters because making the necessary measurements directly from the scan is very convenient. Further, a copy of the scan can be used during surgery to correlate the scan to the patient's bony architecture.

Table 8.3 Treatment factors for dental implant placement.

Need for bone graft (?)
Need for guided bone regeneration graft (?)
Implant design
Need for a custom abutment (?)
Crown selection
Interim partial denture (?)
Implant maintenance

Table 8.4 Implant system selection.

- Tapered
- Bone level
- Internal connection
- Platform switch
- Long-term availability
- Wide array of restorative options
  - Stock abutments (straight/ angled)
  - Engaging/ non engaging
  - UCLA abutments
  - Multi-unit abutments
  - Ti bases
  - Digital scan transfers

The site criteria for a simple implant to be placed from the first molar and forward are indicated in Table 8.2 but are repeated here for emphasis:

- Bone width: ≥6 mm
- Bone height: ≥6 mm
- While the rule of 6 applies to the bone height as an absolute minimum requirement, it is highly recommended to have a 2 mm zone of safety when dealing with the inferior alveolar nerve. So, if placing a 6 mm implant in the posterior mandible, 8 mm of bone height would be needed.
- Inter-occlusal space: ≥6 mm

If the bone criteria are not satisfied, then grafting or guided bone regeneration (GBR) may be necessary. Typical situations where grafting is necessary are discussed in Chapter 9.

The next decision is the choice of the implant system, Table 8.4.

The guidelines for deciding upon an implant choice are indicated in Table 8.5.

We are not advocating that all dentists must use implants with the listed criteria but rather that we have found that a tapered internal connection system (Fig. 8.1) to work the best in our multi-facility group. With so many systems available, dentists should opt for the system that they are most comfortable with and that works best for them. Another factor, of course, is overhead and the various available systems differ in cost, which can be a factor in system selection.

Regardless of the implant system selected, the implant site or the various patient factors, the cautious dentist should always anticipate the worst and prepare for the need for bone grafting regardless of pre-operative radiographic evidence. That is why it is advisable to reflect a full thickness flap for the first 50 or so implant placements until sufficient experience is gained to enable the dentist to readily visualize the implant site prior to surgery. It is also advisable to be prepared to be able to furnish an interim RPD in situations where the patient has concerns over facial appearance after placement of the implant.

Table 8.5   Selection criteria for implant systems.

- Tapered: implants with a taper are safer in critical areas compared to parallel implants
- Bone level: placing at the bone level provides more restorative options compared to tissue level implants
- Internal connection: more retentive system compared to external connections
- Platform switch: the horizontal offset provides better bone stability at the implant-abutment interface compared to flush abutment-implant interfaces
- Long-term availability of the system: Some less well-established systems with unique connections may not be available 10 or 20 years into the future which will create problems if restorative complications arise

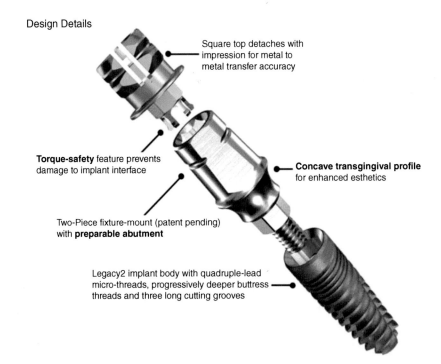

Design Details

Square top detaches with impression for metal to metal transfer accuracy

Torque-safety feature prevents damage to implant interface

Concave transgingival profile for enhanced esthetics

Two-Piece fixture-mount (patent pending) with **preparable abutment**

Legacy2 implant body with quadruple-lead micro-threads, progressively deeper buttress threads and three long cutting grooves

Figure 8.1   Design details of the Legacy 4 system (*Source*: Courtesy of Implant Direct Inc.).

Surgical Procedure

The pre-operative protocol should always incorporate a review of the patient's medical history and recording the blood pressure and pulse rate. This is followed by pre-rinsing with chlorhexidine solution to reduce the bacterial load. Thereafter, the patient should be anesthetized, typically with maxillary infiltration of both the buccal and palatal, and/or a mandibular block.

The surgical procedure for a simple implant is outlined in Table 8.6.

There are two approaches to creating access, namely flap reflection Fig. 8.2a,b, or a surgical punch (flapless), Fig. 8.3.

The advantage of flap reflection is that the surgical site is clearly seen and is readily accessible. Further, it allows the operator to score the bone surface with a surgical drill to accurately position the implant placement, Fig. 8.2b.

Table 8.6 Steps in surgical procedure for a simple implant.

1. Create access
2. Perform osteotomy
3. Place the implant
4. Site closure

(a)   (b)

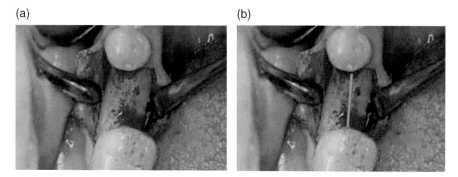

Figure 8.2 (a) Flap reflection to expose the bone. (b) Scoring the cortical bone surface for accurate implant placement.

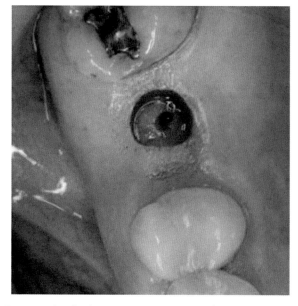

Figure 8.3 Creating alveolar bone access using a punch.

The disadvantage of flap reflection is that the reflected tissue must be sutured back in place after implant insertion.

In contrast, for the more experienced dentist, utilizing a punch to gain access to the cortical bone surface (Fig. 8.3) is simpler. However, whereas the punch approach gets around the need for flap reflection, it does necessitate accurate location of the required osteotomy hole on a first-time basis. Later, this will avoid unnecessary osteotomies to create the correct access, which can cause damage to the otherwise intact bone. The other disadvantage of the tissue punch is the removal of keratinized gingiva. In areas where there is minimal keratinized gingiva, it is advised to utilize a full thickness flap to preserve the tissue.

Performing the Osteotomy

Three basic steps are important in performing the osteotomy regardless of the mode of access:

- Center the osteotomy
- Establish the length of the osteotomy
- Establish the width of the osteotomy.

The surgical steps in preparing the osteotomy (implant placement) site are indicated in Table 8.7.

Complete surgical osteotomy kits are available, Fig. 8.4, which provide all the bone drills and tools for performing an osteotomy.

Surgical Procedure

Step 1: An initial bone incision is made with a locator drill to a depth of 6–8 mm. After taking a radiograph and carrying out analysis to check the accurate positioning of the hole using a locating indicator, the locator drill is then used to drill to the full length (depth) required for the implant, typically 10 mm.

Step 2: The initial osteotomy in soft bone is progressively widened using osteotomy drills of increasing diameter, Fig. 8.5.

Coarser thread and heavier duty drills are used for dense bone, Fig. 8.6.

Table 8.7   Osteotomy procedure.

1. Establish the center of your final restoration
    a. Purchase point made with a high-speed surgical bur
    b. Center B-L, M-D
2. Establish the length (implant depth)
    a. Length is established with locator drill (sharp-tipped drill)
    b. Use radiographs to check angles
    c. The most common implant body length is 10 mm. In the authors' opinion, there are no benefits to exceed a depth of 10 mm in healed bone.
3. Establish the width
    a. Width is based on the width of bone and on the tooth to be restored
       • Anterior 3.2–4.7 mm width
       • Premolar 3.7–4.7 mm width
       • Molar 4.7–7 mm width

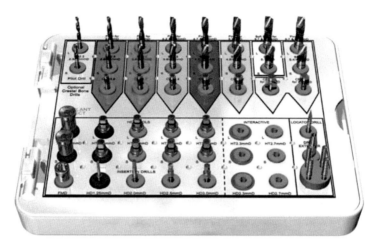

Figure 8.4 Surgical osteotomy kit (*Source*: Courtesy of Implant Direct Inc.).

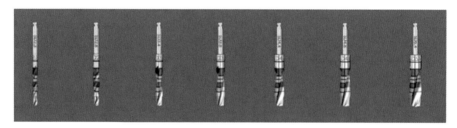

Figure 8.5 Osteotomy soft bone drills of progressively increasing diameter (*Source*: Courtesy of Implant Direct Inc.).

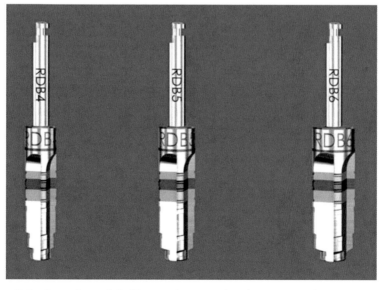

Figure 8.6 Dense bone drills (*Source*: Courtesy of Implant Direct Inc.).

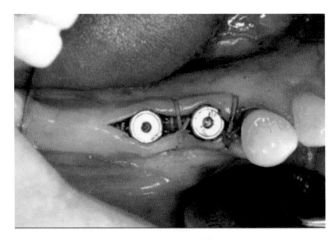

Figure 8.7   Seated healing abutments and sutured flap.

In order to maintain a clean (saliva-free) work site and prevent burning and possible bone necrosis, the osteotomy site should be continuously irrigated with sterile saline solution. Ideally, the osteotomy should be isolated from saliva to prevent contamination.

Step 3: Remove the implant body from its packaging and insert into the prepared site using the provided carrier. After initial placement, torque the implant/carrier in place with the torque driver. Remove the carrier and, after reviewing the positioning and placement, fine tune positioning: *the implant platform should be flush with the bone level or 0.5–1 mm below the bone level.*

Note: The torque wrench should be set to 50 Ncm. If the implant cannot be inserted to the requisite depth (10 mm and at the bone level or 0.5–1 mm below the bone level), back the implant out and use the corresponding dense bone drill to widen the osteotomy. It is important to not over-torque the implant to place.

Step 4: Insert the healing abutment or cover screw with driver to 15 Ncm and suture the reflected flap tissue in place, Fig. 8.7. Note that it is important to maintain the buccal keratinized tissue accomplished at initial flap design.

When suturing the flap, we recommend the use of Cytoplast Polytetrafluoroethylene (PTFE) suture material, Fig. 8.8, since we have found this to be easily handled and it passes through tissue easily without snagging or tearing.

Time-Line for a Simple Implant

1. Surgery
2. Two-week follow-up with radiographs and, if necessary, suture removal.
3. Impressions. These are taken at six to eight weeks post-surgery.
4. Delivery of the crown at 10–12 weeks post-surgery

An example of a simple implant placement to replace a missing tooth is shown in Figs. 8.9 – Fig. 8.13.

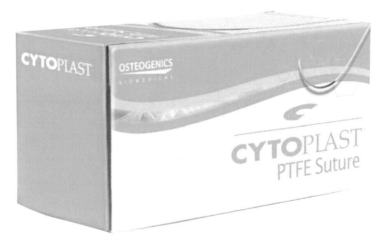

Figure 8.8   Cytoplast PTFE suture (*Source*: Courtesy of Implant Direct).

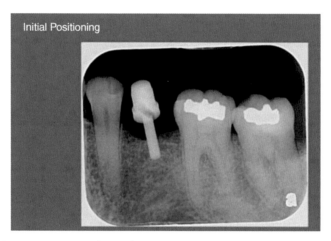

Figure 8.9   Pre-operative radiograph.

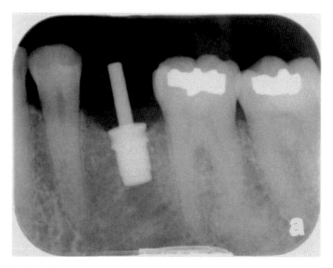

Figure 8.10   Initial positioning.

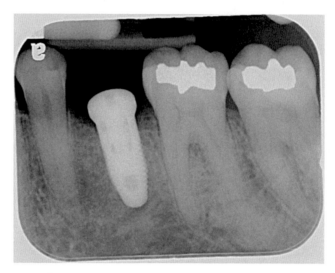

Figure 8.11   Final positioning.

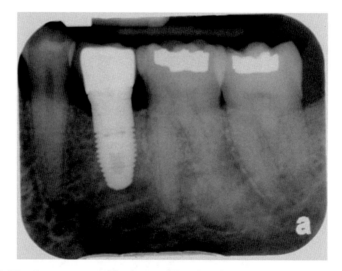

Figure 8.12   Cement retained final restoration placed.

The following case, replacing a failing Maryland bridge, is a step-by-step example of the placement of a simple implant. This step-by-step approach is indicated in Figures 8.14 to 8.17. Note that the Maryland bridge is used as a temporary restoration during the implant healing period.

Post-operative Protocol

1. Eating or other potential trauma to the operative site should be avoided: adjacent teeth may be brushed but not the surgical site for at least 48 hours.
2. Antibiotic may be prescribed, typically Amoxicillin 500 mg, TID, for five to seven days provided the patient is not allergic.

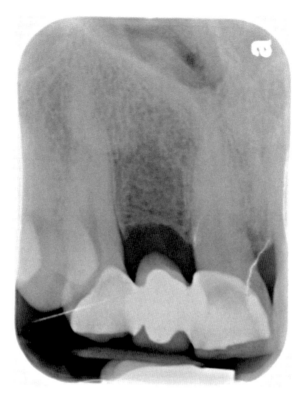

Figure 8.13 Failing Maryland bridge.

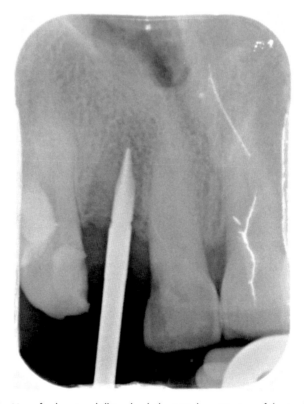

Figure 8.14 Use of a locator drill to check the initial positioning of the implant.

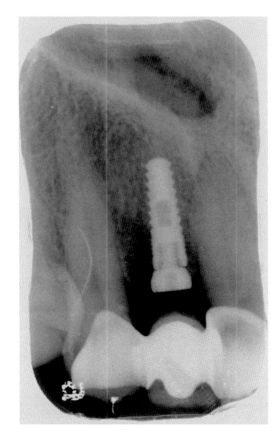

Figure 8.15 Placement of the implant.

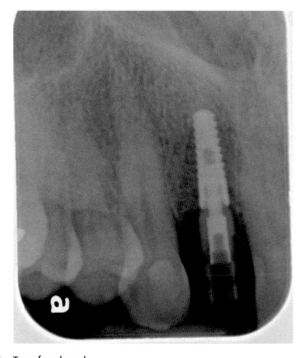

Figure 8.16 Transfer placed.

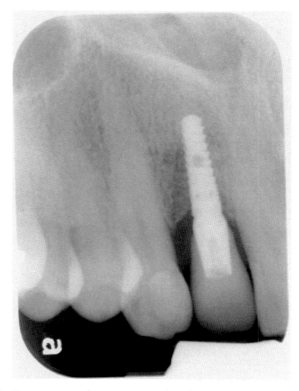

Figure 8.17   Cement retained e.max crown placed.

3. Chlorhexidine rinse BID for 10 days.
4. Warm salt water rinses after meals.
5. Pain medications: recommend or prescribe as determined by the patient medical history. Typically, ibuprofen 600–800 mg is sufficient for most healed site implant placement procedures.
6. Schedule a two-week follow-up appointment.

Conclusions

The most basic surgical requirement for implant placement is having adequate bone volume and quality. The rule of 6's states that the patient should have a minimum of 6 mm of bone in all dimensions as well as 6 mm of interocclusal space. It is the authors' opinion that raising a flap to visualize the bony architecture is recommended for the practitioner's first 50 cases. Performing an osteotomy in healed bone follows a very systematic approach of first creating a purchase point, establishing the osteotomy depth, and finally establishing the osteotomy width. Upon completion of the machining of the osteotomy, the implant is then placed to depth.

Reference

1. Kasat, V. and Ladda, R. (2012). Smoking and dental implants. *J. Int. Soc. Prev. Community Dent.* 2 (2): 38–41.

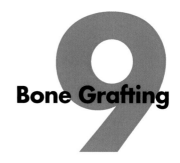

Bone Grafting

Bone regeneration or, simply, pre-implant bone grafting is an important aspect of dental implantology. In fact, bone regeneration is often mandatory following tooth extraction and prior to implant placement, and there are several reasons for this. The successful placement of implants requires sufficient bone volume of high biological quality for the implant to osseointegrate prior to its subsequent restoration. Specifically, the rule of 6's applies where 6 mm of bone is necessary in a vertical and horizontal dimension. When an implant is treatment planned, it is generally because the patient's tooth is deemed non-restorable. This "hopeless" prognosis is reached based on several factors including caries at or below the bone level, failing endodontic treatment, perio-endo lesions, advanced periodontal disease, and tooth fracture. All of these conditions potentially affect the underlying hard and soft tissue.

Other factors necessitating bone grafting include post-extraction resorption of the edentulous ridge, the presence of bony defects due to trauma or infection as well as the need to place implants in specific sites for proper functionality. Further, in esthetic areas, a satisfactory emergence profile of the soft tissue requires a bony base because it is well-established that soft tissue follows its hard tissue base. Finally, in situations where there has been significant loss of bone and the tooth is deemed unsalvageable, guided bone regeneration (GBR) is used to facilitate bone regeneration when the bone thickness in the jaw is insufficient for implant placement.

In other words, bone grafting or GBR has two primary purposes:

- To meet the criteria of bone volume for implant placement, or
- To improve the results of an implant prosthesis by allowing a more ideal position of the implant.

The ADA Practical Guide to Dental Implants, First Edition. Luigi O. Massa and J. Anthony von Fraunhofer.
© 2021 The American Dental Association. Published 2021 by John Wiley & Sons, Inc.

(a)   (b)

(c)   (d)

(e)

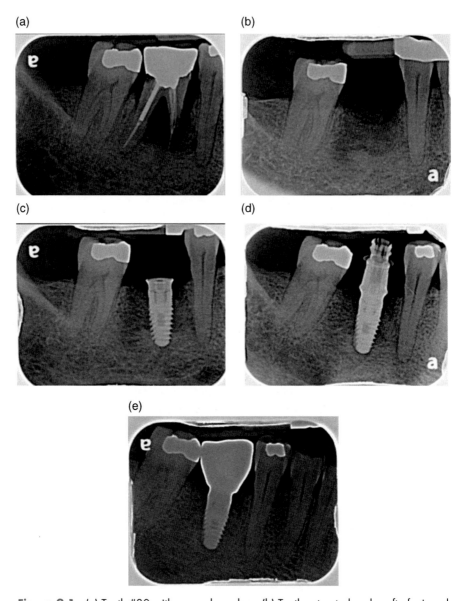

Figure 9.1 (a) Tooth #30 with severe bone loss. (b) Tooth extracted and graft of mineralized cortico-cancellous bone placed with a non-resorbing membrane. (c) Implant placed five months post-GBR. (d) Implant level impression. (e) Final restoration.

A typical example of a situation requiring GBR is shown in Figs. 9.1a,b,c,d,e, covering the replacement of a "hopeless" situation with tooth #30.

The basic rules of bone grafting in an extraction site with a wall defect (generally, the defect will occur on the buccal plate) are the following:

1. Raise a flap to visualize the defect.
2. Carefully curette all granulation tissue out of the socket and create blood flow.
3. Irrigate with sterile saline.

4. Place barrier membrane along defect.
5. Place bone graft material.
6. Close site with
   a. Primary closure which entails advancement of the flap to cover the graft – a resorbable or non-resorbable membrane can be utilized. If a non-resorbable membrane is utilized, it must be retrieved at the time of re-entry.
   b. Secondary closure – a non-resorbable membrane is generally utilized to "cover" the graft. Generally, the non-resorbable membranes are made to withstand the acids and enzymes in the oral cavity.

Bone Grafting

Graft materials are discussed in detail in Appendix C but for convenience, a few comments are made here. There are basically four classes of material utilized for GBR:

- An allograft – a tissue graft from a donor of the same species as the recipient but not genetically identical.
- An autograft – a graft of tissue harvested from the patient, e.g., bone harvested from the iliac crest or patella plane for gap filling or sinus lifting.
- A xenograft – tissue harvested from a species other than human.
- Synthetic graft material.

Theoretically, autografting is the optimal approach to bone grafting but, as this procedure usually involves an ancillary surgical procedure to harvest the bone, it is not the preferred approach despite certain inherent advantages. The first of these advantages is that there is no need for sterilization or sanitization of the graft material. Second, the risk of rejection by the recipient site is minimized although it must be borne in mind that once bone is harvested from the donor site and separated from its vascular supply, that bone may die before it can heal. Although rejection is uncommon, it can still occur because the transplanted material will be "foreign" to the recipient site.

Similar considerations regarding rejection apply to allografting and xenografting. In both cases, sanitization/sterilization is necessary to ensure a pristine and bacteria-free implantation. On the other hand, the advantage of both these approaches is that the particle sizing of the grafting materials and their sanitization/sterilization are performed prior to their use, and they are commercially available. As noted, graft materials are discussed in detail in Appendix C.

Regarding the selection of a graft material, the general consensus is:

- Survival rates of implants placed into grafted areas are comparable with survival rates of implants placed into pristine bone [1].
- Bone quality at the recipient site determines the type of graft material to be used. Cortical bone is inferior to cancellous bone at the recipient bed. Cells within cancellous bone are responsible for at least 60% of bone healing capacity. The periosteum in a young, healthy patient contributes an additional 30% whereas cells in cortical bone only contribute about 10% to overall bone healing.

When bone resorbs after extraction, the cancellous bone shrinks relative to cortical bone. As the cancellous component of the jawbone diminishes, there is a corresponding decreasing in the reservoir for osteoblasts. However, computerized tomography (CT) can indicate the ratio of cancellous to cortical bone at the recipient site prior to surgery, this ratio facilitating graft material selection as follows:

1. Only cortical bone: autograft.
2. Cortico-cancellous bone: selection depends on which predominates but if there is a preponderance of cancellous bone, the choice is less critical.

Ridge Preservation

There is strong clinical evidence that ridge preservation techniques are usually effective in limiting post-extraction horizontal and vertical bone loss when compared to healing that relies solely on a blood clot. In fact, ridge preservation significantly maintains ridge width and height (refer to Figs. 9.1a,b,c,d,e). The prevailing opinion is that most graft materials are effective for this purpose with only slight differences being found between them.

"External" augmentation procedures, regardless of whether they are horizontal or vertical, on the alveolar ridge are more difficult than "internal" augmentation in areas like the maxillary sinus. The consensus is that augmentations of vertical alveolar ridge defects generally have lower rates of successful healing outcomes than those for horizontal defects. However, for both horizontal and vertical ridge augmentation procedures, the use of autogenous bone blocks appear to result in greater bone gain than found with particulate allograft materials. The good thing is that the survival rates of implants placed in well-healed horizontally and vertically augmented alveolar ridges are high.

It should be noted that whereas autogenous onlay bone-grafting procedures performed to allow implant placement are effective and predictable for the correction of severely resorbed edentulous ridges, survival rates are somewhat lower than those of implants placed into pristine bone.

The confounding factors regarding implant survival in grafted sites include:

• Poor blood supply, trauma, or extensive surgery in the area, all of which adversely affect the implant prognosis.
• Post-surgical complications and poor implant prognoses are higher in smokers.
• General diseases that affect bone metabolism, e.g., uncontrolled diabetes, head and neck radiation and bisphosphonate therapy, appear to be relative contraindications for bone augmentation or at least may be somewhat predictive of long-term implant failure.

Membranes

GBR is commonly used in combination with membranes during implant placement, the primary purpose being to exclude non-osteogenic tissues from interfering with bone regeneration following GBR therapy.

Many types of membrane have been introduced for both experimental and clinical application (see Appendix C). This development has led to many research and clinical papers regarding the properties and biological outcomes with different membranes [2]. Membranes are usually provided with a porous structure but the optimal porosity and, indeed, the precise role of membrane porosity in the barrier function of GBR membranes is still uncertain. It appears, however, that in addition to providing a barrier function, membranes may actively participate in the regenerative processes occurring within the defect during GBR.

The clinician about to place a membrane has to decide between resorbable and non-resorbable materials, and several factors come into play in this decision, Table 9.1.

Table 9.1 Selection of barrier membranes.

Factor	Resorbable	Non-resorbable
Cost	Higher cost	Less costly
Longevity in situ	4–6 months	Permanent
Retrievability	Unnecessary	Retrieval necessary

At this time, it is unknown whether resorbable or non-resorbable membranes have better clinical properties and performance. However, because the bone graft ideally should be left undisturbed for four to six months in order to achieve the most predictable pre-implant bone regeneration, then using resorbable membranes and eliminating the need to remove a non-resorbable membrane might appear to be sensible. It is important to note that it may be preferable to achieve primary closure over a membrane because membrane exposure in general has a higher complication rate [3].

GBR Clinical Sequence

Fig. 9.2 shows a common clinical situation where GBR is necessary to provide a satisfactory implant site.

Step 1. Elevate flap using releasing incisions (Fig. 9.3)
Step 2. Decorticate deficient bone plate to increase blood supply to graft (Fig. 9.4)
Step 3. Place membrane (e.g., cytoplast resorbable regenerative tissue matrix (RTM)/Kontour™).
Step 4. Place graft material (e.g., Directgen™ mineralized cortico-cancellous particulate)
Step 5. Suture implant site using non-traumatic sutures (e.g., cytoplast PTFE non-resorbable) with tension-free closure (Fig. 9.5).

The clinical application of the above procedures is shown in Figs. 9.6 – Fig. 9.9.

Crestal Sinus Augmentation

Another common clinical situation is the need for crestal sinus augmentation, i.e., when the proposed implant site does not satisfy the requirement of 6 mm minimum vertical bone height

(a)

(c)

(b)

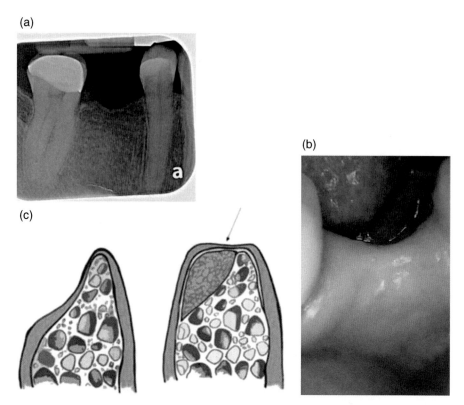

Figure 9.2 (a) and (b) Radiograph and clinical photograph of a narrow ridge. (c) Schematic diagram of a narrow bone ridge requiring GBR prior to implant placement.

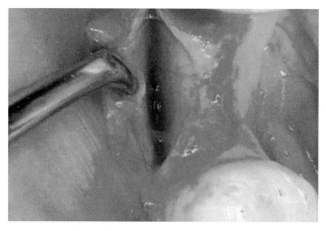

Figure 9.3 Reflecting a flap.

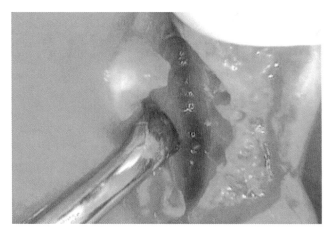

Figure 9.4 Decorticated deficient buccal plate.

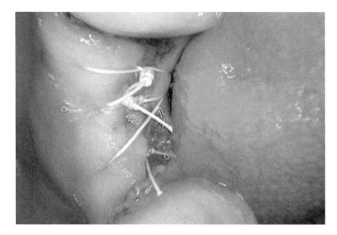

Figure 9.5 Suture flap after membrane and graft placement.

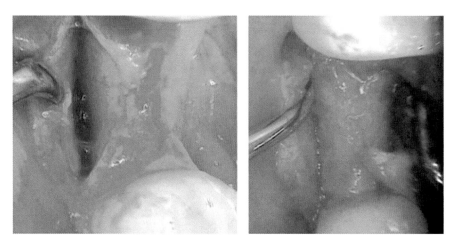

Figure 9.6 Clinical situation before and after 9 months of healing.

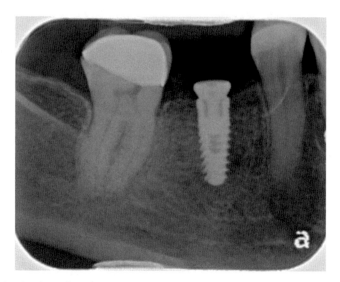

Figure 9.7 Implant placed.

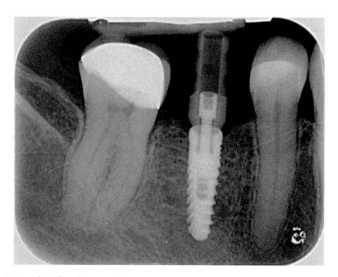

Figure 9.8 Implant level impression.

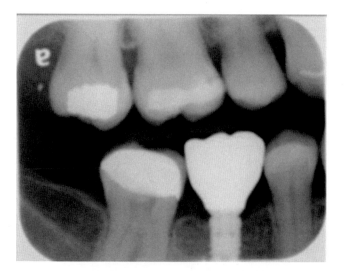

Figure 9.9 Final screw-retained restoration placed.

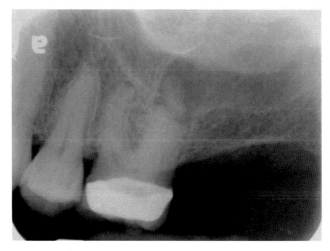

Figure 9.10 Fractured root #14.

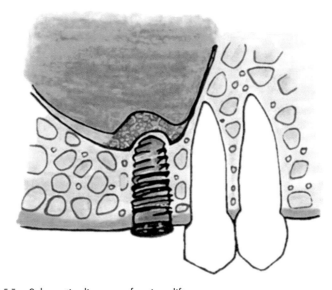

Figure 9.11 Schematic diagram of a sinus lift.

Step 1. Establish bone height with pilot drill and radiographs – note that the cortical bone of the sinus floor "feels" different than the soft medullary bone of the posterior maxilla.

Step 2. Trephine to the established bone height.

Step 3. Fracture the cortical floor (Fig. 9.11).

Step 4 (with the example shown in Fig. 9.10) with an extraction site and osteotomy as seen in Fig. 9.12:

Step 5. Close-up of sinus membrane (Fig. 9.13).

Step 6. Place implant (Fig. 9.14a).

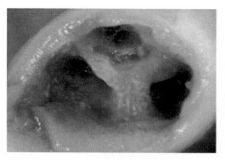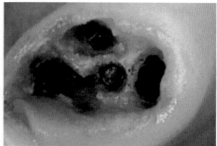

Figure 9.12 Extraction site and osteotomy.

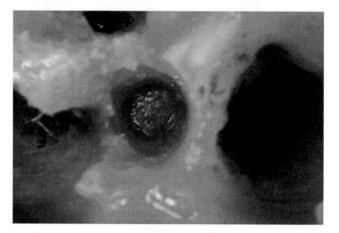

Figure 9.13 Close-up of sinus membrane.

Note

The appropriate codes for insurance reimbursement (when applicable) for GBR therapy prior to implant placement are:

D6104: Bone graft at time of implant placement
D7953: Socket preservation
D4266: GBR resorbable
D4267: GBR non resorbable

It is also of the greatest importance that the clinician addresses the following when planning any form of implant placement with or without bone grafting:

a. Provide the patient with a clear and concise presentation regarding the intended procedures and the reasons underlying the proposed treatment.
b. An educated patient will not only be more compliant and motivated, but also be an enthusiastic source of referrals.
c. Ensure that the patient clearly understands the procedures involved and their cost, i.e. provide the patient with a clear and simple price structure.
d. Train staff regarding both the implant procedure and the need and desire to provide optimal patient care.

(a)

(b)

(c)

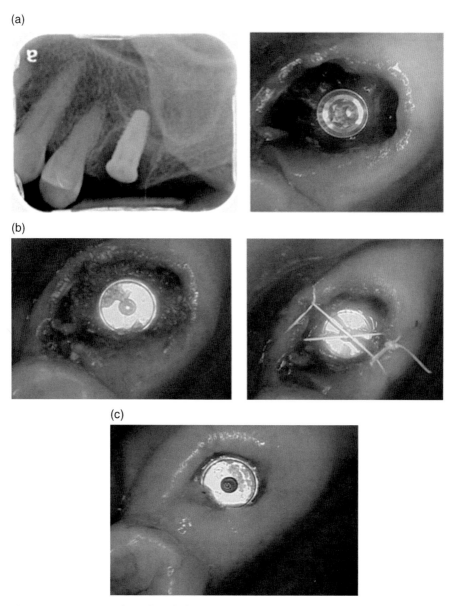

Figure 9.14 (a) Implant placed. (b) Implant grafted and sutured. (c) Two-week follow-up after suture removal. (d) Impressing the implant. (e) 12-month post-operative radiograph.

(d)

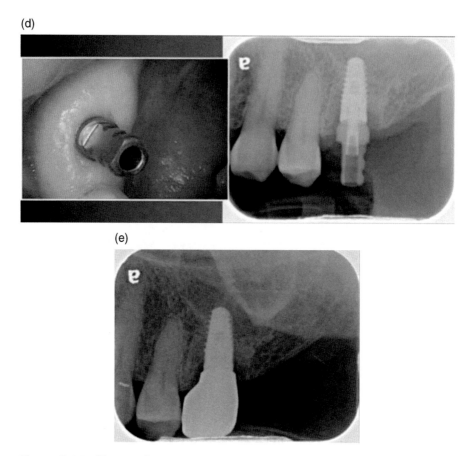

(e)

Figure 9.14 (Continued)

Conclusions

In Implant Dentistry, bone grafting is used to develop or enhance the potential surgical site. Socket preservation is performed at the time of extraction to develop the site for future implant placement. If there is a wall defect, barrier membranes are used to retard epithelial ingrowth into the graft material. The sinus can be augmented either vertically through the osteotomy or horizontally through a lateral wall to increase bone volume for implant placement. The mastery of grafting techniques allows nearly all sites to have the potential for implant placement.

References

1. Duong, T.T., Gay, I., Diaz-Rodriguez, J. et al. (2016). Survival of dental implants placed in grafted and non-grafted bone: a retrospective study in a university setting. *Int. J. Oral Maxillofac. Implants* 31 (2): 310–317.
2. Elgali, I., Omar, O., Dahlin, C., and Thomsen, P. (2017). Guided bone regeneration: materials and biological mechanisms revisited. *Eur. J. Oral Sci.* 125: 315–337.
3. Machtei, E.E. (2001). The effect of membrane exposure on the outcome of regenerative procedures in humans: a meta-analysis. *J. Periodontol.* 72 (4): 512–516.

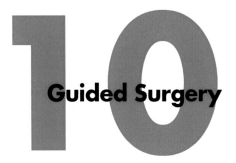

Guided Surgery

For as long as dental surgeons have been placing implants, there have been continuous advancements and innovations. One of the areas where innovation has flourished is in *guided implant surgery*. Early implant planning consisted of 2D radiography and bone sounding, requiring clinicians to visualize structures by reflecting flaps. Accordingly, early implant surgery tended to be unpredictable because of the many unknowns involved in the procedure.

Restorative guides have been extensively used during implant planning and placement. A restorative-based guide is a pattern or template that will aid the surgeon in visualizing the proposed position of the final restorations. An example would be a clear duplicate denture or an acrylic "suck-down" of a mocked-up tooth on a model, (Figs. 10.1 and 10.2). One major problem with a restorative guide is that the restorative goals and the bony architecture do not always match up; a situation that can render the guide ineffective and create a restorative compromise.

Imaging

Radiography has been a mainstay in dentistry since the mid-1900s, and X-rays are an effective way of finding, and identifying, various oral problems. Although ubiquitous, the information discernible from a conventional radiograph can be limited and lack precision regarding the location of abnormalities and lesions which can present problems when planning implant dentistry.

Greater radiologic precision became possible with the introduction of X-ray computed tomography (CT), also known as computerized tomographic imaging or computerized axial tomography (CAT) [1–4]. This diagnostic imaging method

The ADA Practical Guide to Dental Implants, First Edition. Luigi O. Massa and J. Anthony von Fraunhofer.
© 2021 The American Dental Association. Published 2021 by John Wiley & Sons, Inc.

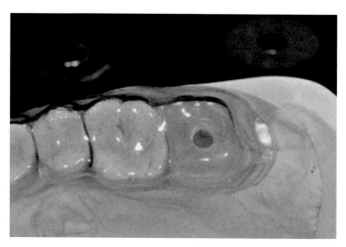

Figure 10.1   Restorative acrylic "suck-down" single tooth guide.

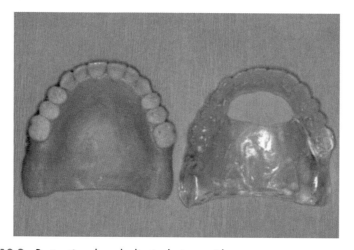

Figure 10.2   Restorative clear duplicate denture guide.

is now considered by the American Academy of Oral and Maxillofacial Radiology to be one of the parameters of care in dental implant planning [5].

In fact, there are two categories of X-ray CT and they differ in their modes of acquiring imaging data based on their respective X-ray beam geometries although both use a low-dose beam of X-rays. These two modalities or categories are *fan beam X-Ray* CT and *Cone Beam Computed Tomography* (CBCT).

In fan-beam scanners, a narrow fan-shaped X-ray beam is projected through the patient's head and collected by a single scanner/detector mounted in the same axial plane as the X-ray source but on the opposite side of the stabilized patient head. Thus, the X-ray source and detector move synchronously around the patient's head. In operation, images are taken slice-by-slice and these images are then "stacked" by sophisticated computer software and processed to produce a detailed 2D cross-sectional image of the head at a greater precision than possible with conventional radiographs [3]. Further, modern imaging systems use multi-detector arrays so that scanning times are markedly reduced, and considerably lower X-ray dosages are used compared to single detector fan-beam CT systems. Further, 3D images are possible with such modern instrumentation.

In contrast to fan-beam CT, CBCT systems are based on volumetric tomography using a divergent or cone-shaped, i.e., a 3D incident X-ray beam. During operation, the CBCT system performs a single 360° scan in which the X-ray source and a reciprocating area detector synchronously move around the patient's head. At certain degree intervals, single projection images, known as "basis" images, are acquired by the detector system. These images are similar to lateral cephalometric radiographic images but each is slightly offset from the next; the series of basis projection images is referred to as the projection data. Thereafter, the system software uses these image data to generate a 3D volumetric data set which, in turn, is used to provide reconstruction images in three orthogonal planes (axial, sagittal, and coronal).

The introduction of CBCT in dentistry was a huge advance in dental implant planning, enabling the surgeon to visualize structures in three dimensions. Practitioners created techniques to fabricate CBCT radiographic guides. Early CBCT scanners were extremely expensive and making a CBCT radiographic guide was relatively labor and technology intensive because trying to make the CBCT data useful in surgery was complicated. It often involved fabricating an appliance with radio-opaque markers that had to be used while taking the CBCT. Despite claims to the contrary, these guides, at best, were only aides to placing implants because they lacked precision and had limited accuracy.

The technology available today allows a streamlined and seamless workflow to create extremely precise surgical guides. There is an array of software which makes this possible. The software will merge the data from a CBCT (digital imaging and communications in medicine [DICOM] data file) with the data from a scanned arch or scanned model (stereolithography [STL] data file). These merged data allow the clinician to visualize the bony architecture in relation to the teeth and soft tissues. The software can also "mock-up" the proposed restoration and map out critical structures such as the inferior alveolar nerve, enabling the clinician to perform "virtual surgery".

Virtual surgery consists of utilizing all the information available to perform surgery on the software. This includes selecting the implant size and the implant orientation in its optimal position. Figs. 10.3 – Fig. 10.7 illustrate virtual surgery in action.

A surgical guide is designed based on the virtual surgery. The surgical guide is made to fit the scanned arch or scanned model. The surgical guide is manufactured utilizing a 3D printer (Fig. 10.8) or by milling out the guide from an acrylic resin. Implant companies have metallic sleeves which correspond to drill kits that are inserted into the surgical guide. The guide can then be sterilized and used for surgery.

Figs. 10.9 and Fig. 10.10 illustrate the virtual surgery process and the actual surgical results when the outlined procedure is followed.

Guided implant surgery has changed dental implantology. It allows clinicians to precisely plan implant placement in all three dimensions. Its primary advantage is that both greater precision and enhanced protection of vital structures are possible because the clinician can now accommodate, anticipate, and avoid vital structures and bony architecture.

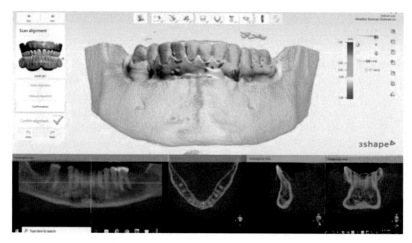

Figure 10.3 Data merge: the CBCT is merged with a scanned arch or scanned model. (*Source:* 3Shape A/S).

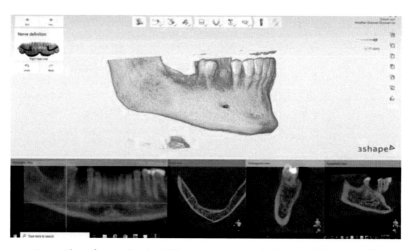

Figure 10.4 The inferior alveolar (IA) nerve is mapped. (*Source:* 3Shape A/S).

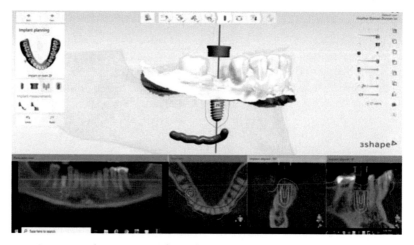

Figure 10.5 Virtual surgery is performed. (*Source:* 3Shape A/S).

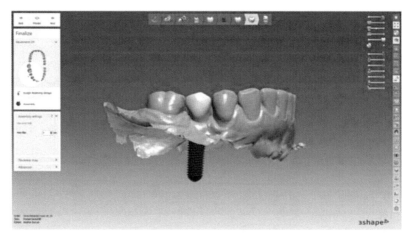

Figure 10.6 Virtual surgery in relation to planned prosthesis. (*Source:* 3Shape A/S).

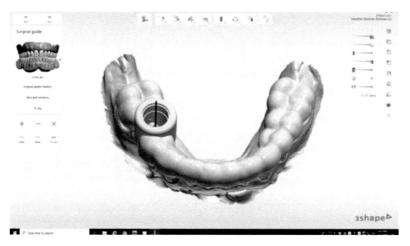

Figure 10.7 Surgical guide design. (*Source:* 3Shape A/S).

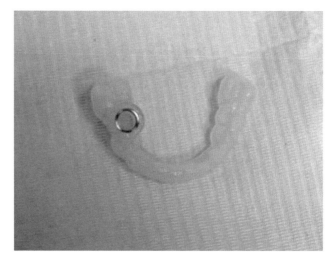

Figure 10.8 3D Printed surgical guide.

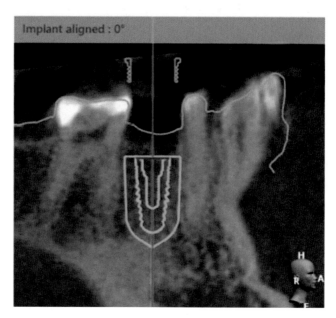

Figure 10.9 Virtual surgery.

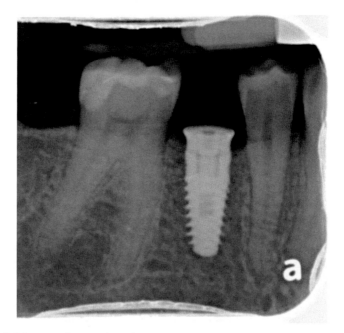

Figure 10.10 Actual surgical results.

Not only is guided implant surgery of major advantage to the clinician but there are also several benefits for the patient, notably:

- Faster surgery
- Less post-operative swelling due to minimizing the need for flap reflection
- Safer surgery due to avoidance of all critical structures.

The time and energy involved in the clinician becoming familiar with the new technology as well as the financial investment in this technology will be amply repaid over time because:

a. Surgery is safer, potentially more accurate and faster
b. There is greater precision in implant planning and placement
c. Implant restoration is more precise with improved esthetics
d. Patients appreciate the reduced surgical time, reduced pain and greater safety
e. Reduced stress on the patient.

Conclusions

Surgical guides are aides to help improve clinical outcomes in implant dentistry. Standard 2D radiographs (Panoramic radiographs and peri-apical radiographs) only allow the practitioner to view the bone in two dimensions – mesial-distally and vertically. CBCT use in dentistry allows the clinician to see the complete bony architecture in all three dimensions – mesial-distally, vertically, and horizontally. The modern surgical planning software merges the CBCT 3D radiograph with a stone cast or intraoral scan of the teeth and soft tissue. This allows for a precise restorative-driven implant plan. A surgical guide is then printed to guide the osteotomy.

References

1. Hsich, J. (2003). *Computed Tomography: Principles, Design, Artifacts, and Recent Advances. SPIE Monographs.* Bellingham, WA: Society of Photo-Optical Instrumentation Engineers.
2. Kalender, W.A. (2006). X-ray computed tomography. *Phys. Med. Biol.* 15 (13): R29–R43.
3. Sukovic, P. (2003). Cone beam computed tomography in craniofacial imaging. *Orthod. Craniofac. Res.* 6 (1): 31–36.
4. Scarfe, W.C., Farman, A.G., and Sukovic, P. (2006). Clinical applications of cone-beam computed tomography in dental practice. *J. Can. Dent. Assoc.* 72 (1): 75–80.
5. White, S.C., Heslop, E.W., Hollender, I.G. et al. (2001). Parameters of radiologic care: an official report of the American Academy of Oral and Maxillofacial Radiology. *Oral Surg. Oral Med. Oral Pathol. Oral Radiol. Endod.* 91 (5): 498–511.

11

Complicated Implant Placement: Immediate Sites

Immediate implant placement is the process of placing the endosseous implant immediately after tooth/root removal. Delayed implant placement allows for healing of the extraction site with or without grafting for a period of four to six months. Clinicians should consider immediate implant placement when faced with the overwhelming need to address certain clinical problems. The instances include but are not limited to:

- A failing endodontic treatment
- A hopeless periodontal condition
- A non-restorable tooth
- Tooth loss or severe damage due to trauma.

Some typical emergencies that merit immediate implants can be seen in Fig. 11.1.

Table 11.1 outlines the rationale(s) underlying the decision by both clinician and patient to undertake immediate implant placement in order to address the clinical problems indicated above:

Nevertheless, certain criteria must be satisfied if the case in question is to be satisfactorily resolved and the following requirements are recommended for predictable success:

- Atraumatic extraction of the affected tooth
- Intact buccal and palatal/lingual plates
- Absence of purulence and active infection
- Satisfactory oral and systemic health
- Initial implant stability of 30 N.cm insertion torque

The ADA Practical Guide to Dental Implants, First Edition. Luigi O. Massa and J. Anthony von Fraunhofer.
© 2021 The American Dental Association. Published 2021 by John Wiley & Sons, Inc.

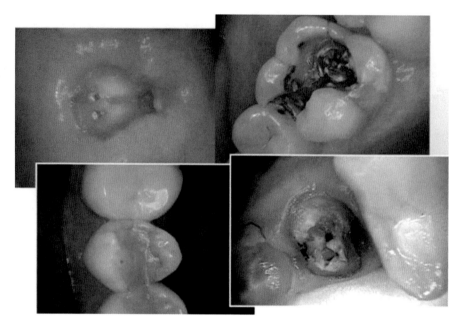

Figure 11.1   Typical dental emergencies that merit immediate implant placement.

Table 11.1   Rationales for immediate implant placement.

Predictable outcome
High acceptance and patient satisfaction
One surgery vs two or three procedures
A fixed temporary restoration can be placed when indicated
Fewer scheduled appointments
Less time elapsed before final restoration (typically 3–4 months)

If the case does not satisfy any of these requirements, then **placement should be delayed** until remedial action has taken effect, as noted above in footnote (a).

Two examples of the need for an implant to treat a failed endodontic restoration and periodontally-involved tooth with severe bone loss [1] are shown in Fig. 11.2 and Fig. 11.3.

In both cases, the size of the bony defects necessitated bone grafting to heal the defects. Consequently, immediate implant placement should not be performed until the defect sites had healed following bone grafting and bony restoration was complete.

There are, of course, several factors that will impact the success (or failure) of the immediately placed implant even when the above criteria are satisfied. The same factors and surgical considerations also apply to delayed placement implants, as discussed elsewhere in this book (Chapters 4, 6–8). Two of the most important of these success-determining factors are the absence of purulence and infection, together with the need for enough sound bone surrounding the osteotomy site in which the implant will be placed. Another important facet of successful immediate implant placement is to ensure primary stability.

It is also important during preparation of the implant cavity that there is minimal trauma to the surrounding bone which, at least in part, depends on avoiding

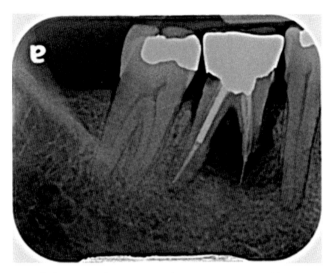

Figure 11.2 Failed root canal treatment with root resorption and bone loss.

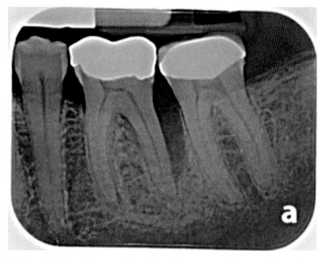

Figure 11.3 Tooth #19 with periodontal involvement and severe bone loss.

excessive heat generation during surgical drilling. Achieving this means that there must be careful control of the force applied and the rotational speed of the osteotomy drill, the design of the drill bit, the drill-bone contact area during the osteotomy **and** there must be effective saline irrigation throughout the surgical procedure.

Steps in placing an immediate implant are as follows:

a. Raise a flap if necessary
b. Create a purchase point with a sharp-end cutting drill slightly favoring the palatal/lingual to compensate for increased buccal bone loss
c. Undersize the osteotomy by 1 drill size to achieve primary stability
d. Place the implant palatal/lingual of center, avoiding contact with the buccal plate

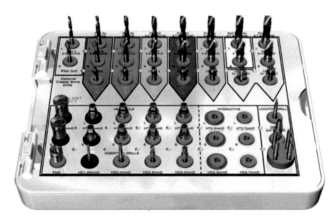

Figure 11.4 A typical oral surgery/implant surgery tool kit (*Source:* Courtesy of Implant Direct Inc.).

e. Place implant at 1–2 mm below the bone crest
f. Graft the gap with demineralized cortico/cancellous particulate bone
g. Do not attempt primary closure

Raising a flap after extraction is discouraged only if the plates can be inspected from the extraction socket. Raising a flap will lead to an increase in bone loss with a thin buccal plate. A purchase point is created to allow subsequent drills to remain centered. Drills will generally take the path of least resistance which can lead to improper positioning. Since immediate implant placement rarely results in the implant being completed encompassed in bone, it is recommended to undersize the osteotomy to increase torque of insertion and improve primary stability. For example: if placing a 4.7 mm diameter implant, one would use the 4.2 mm drill as the final drill in the osteotomy sequence. If the implant does not easily follow the intended insertion path and falls into the extraction socket, it may be necessary to upsize at least the upper half of the implant osteotomy.

Note that many implant manufacturers supply complete surgical tool kits designed for use with their implants, which greatly simplifies the osteotomy and implant placement procedures, Fig. 11.4.

Treatment Sequence

1. Surgery (Extraction/Implant placement)
2. Two-week follow-up
3. Tissue sculpting, if necessary using a temporary restoration or a custom healing abutment
4. Fabrication and placement of the final screw-retained restoration
5. Long-term follow-up

Implant Placement

Ideally, when placing an immediate implant, the fixture should be placed about 1–2 mm below the buccal plate, Fig. 11.5:

In summary, the optimal implant placement positions are the following:

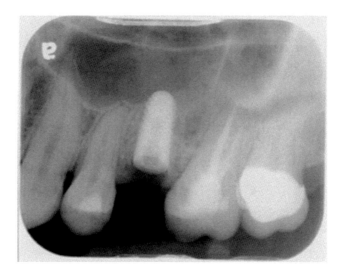

Figure 11.5   Placement of an immediate implant 2 mm below crest of the buccal plate.

- Ideally, 2 mm beyond the apex of the extraction socket if room exists
- For maxillary anteriors: placement into palatal bone and along the palatal wall
- For premolars: placement along the palatal/lingual wall
- For posteriors: placement should be centered mesial-distally and offset toward the palatal/lingual in the inter-septal bone

  Optimal results are achieved when the clinician adheres to the following:

- Utilizes a "locator drill" to create a purchase point and to direct the osteotomy
- Keeps the implant positioned palatally/lingually
- Does not have the implant touch the buccal plate

  In cases when there is a difficult extraction, it may be helpful to create an osteotomy while removing the tooth since this approach will create space to elevate the roots. An example of this approach is shown in Figs. 11.7 – 11.10, a failed restoration of tooth #18:

Immediate Temporization

Immediate temporization has been mentioned several times with regard to the immediate implant. There are at least two important benefits from this approach, the first being maintenance of the soft tissue profile, as shown in clinical photos and radiographs, Figs. 11.6a,b,c. A second radiographic example of the maintenance of emergence profile is shown in Figs. 11.11a,b,c.

The second benefit of immediate temporization is that the patient is provided with a fixed provisional restoration, as shown in Figs. 11.12 – 11.14.

It must be borne in mind that, with any temporization, to minimize deleterious occlusal or masticatory effects on the implant or its bony socket, the temporary be non-functional and out of occlusion. The patient is to be made aware to use extreme caution with the temporary.

(a)

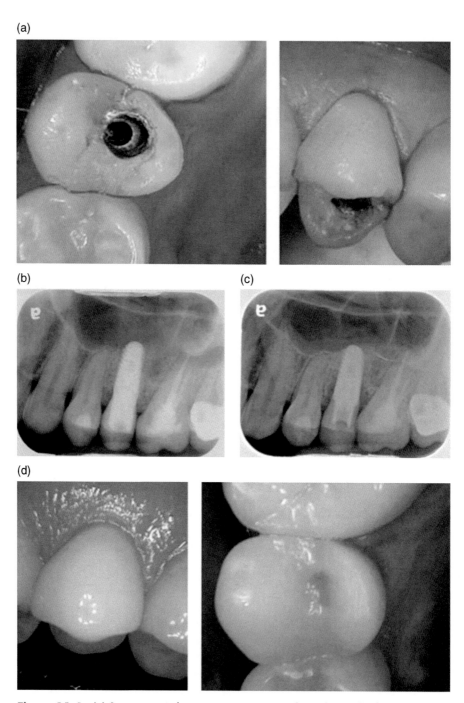

(b)

(c)

(d)

Figure 11.6 (a) Screw-retained temporary restoration. (b) Radiograph of screw-retained temporary restoration. (c) Radiograph of screw-retained e-max final restoration. (d) Restored immediate implant with screw-retained e-max restoration.

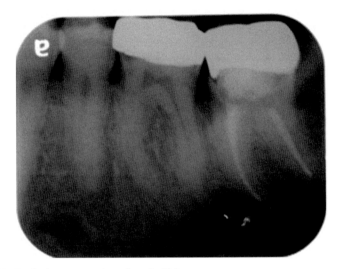

Figure 11.7 Failing restoration of tooth #18.

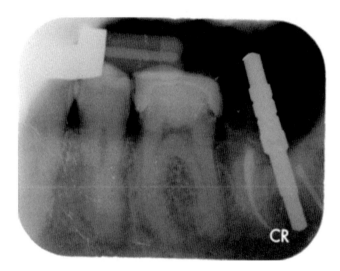

Figure 11.8 Osteotomy created to facilitate extraction.

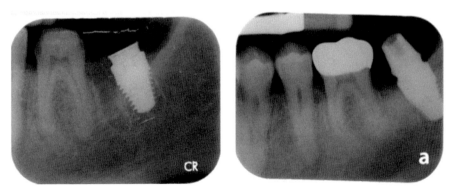

Figure 11.9 Implant placement and impression taking.

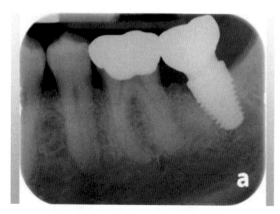

Figure 11.10 Screw-retained zirconia crown.

(a)

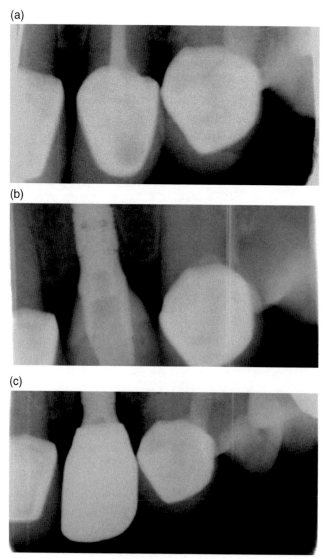

(b)

(c)

Figure 11.11 (a) Original emergence. (b) Immediately loaded temporary restoration. (c) Final restoration.

(a)   (b)

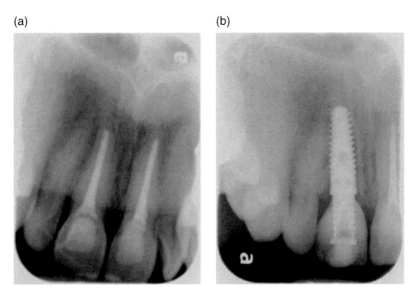

Figure 11.12   Showing (a) and (b) Replacement of a fractured tooth root and temporary restoration.

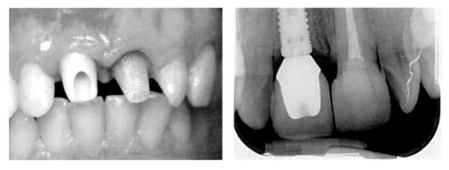

Figure 11.13   Zirconia custom abutment and final e.max restorations.

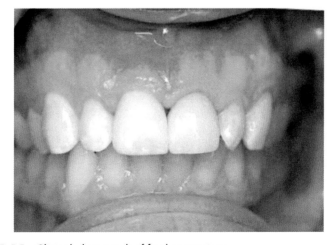

Figure 11.14   Clinical photograph of final restorations.

(a)   (b)

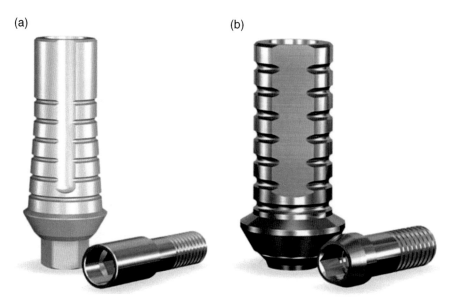

Figure 11.15 (a) PEEK temporary abutment, (b) Titanium temporary abutment (*Source*: Courtesy of Implant Direct).

Types of Temporary Restorations

In the context of temporization of immediate implants, temporary (or provisional) restorations fall into two categories: screw-retained and cement-retained provisionals (see Chapter 13).

Our preferred approach is to use a titanium/plastic temporary abutment to fabricate a screw-retained provisional restoration. We adopt this approach because it permits tissue sculpting and eliminates the need for a cement or luting agent to retain the restoration.

Our protocol for a screw-retained provisional restoration is the following:

1. Template for the provisional restoration is fabricated (pre-operative impression).
2. Set the temporary abutment (Fig. 11.15) into implant but do not screw in.
3. Temporary abutment is "picked up" with temporary material.
4. The emergence profile should be adjusted with flowable composite.
5. Screw hole opened.
6. Screw-retained temporary tried in and adjusted.
7. Torque screw-retained temporary abutment to 15 N.cm.
8. Fill screw access hole with cotton pellet and composite resin.

Figs. 11.16 and Fig. 11.17 are radiographs showing this technique.

Wide-Body Implants

There are certain clinical situations when implants with a greater diameter, so-called wide-body implants, are used in preference to standard implants. These fixtures are especially useful for dealing with four situations in particular:

(a)   (b)

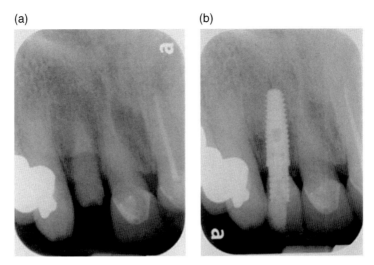

Figure 11.16 (a) Radiograph of failed restoration, (b) Implant placed with Ti temporary abutment and temporary material "picked up".

(a)   (b)

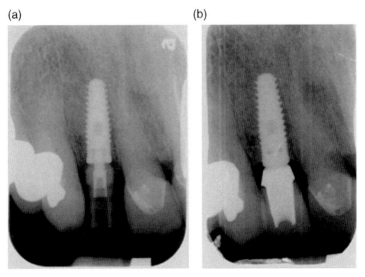

Figure 11.17 (a) Radiograph of the transfer in place, (b) Final zirconia abutment and e.max restoration.

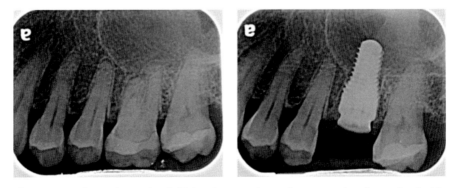

Figure 11.18 Radiograph of #14 with vertical root fracture and radiograph of wide diameter implant placed.

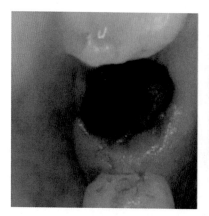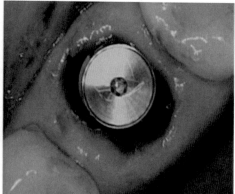

Figure 11.19 Osteotomy site and implant fixture placement.

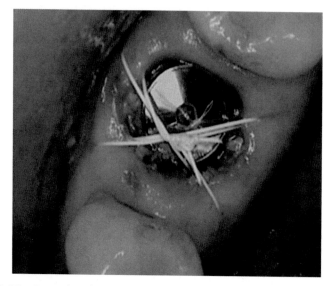

Figure 11.20 Sutured implant site.

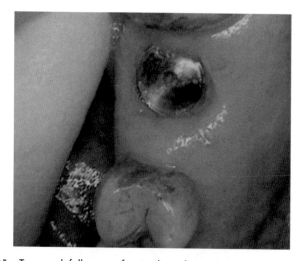

Figure 11.21 Two week follow-up after implant placement.

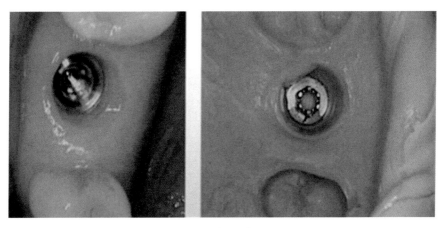

Figure 11.22   Tissue healing at eight weeks and Legacy 4 impression.

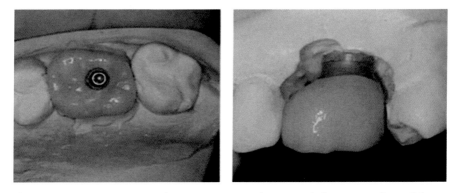

Figure 11.23   Screw-retained zirconia crown with Legacy 4 abutment used as a Ti-base.

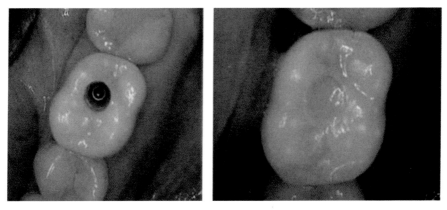

Figure 11.24   Screw-retained zirconia crown delivered with a Legacy 4 abutment used as a Ti-base.

- The tooth to be replaced has a "converging root formation." Molar converging roots will create a large extraction socket upon extraction. This necessitates a larger diameter implant body to gain primary stability.
- There is a need for enhanced initial stability.
- Achieving the optimal emergence profile for molar restorations.
- The anticipated future occlusal forces are above average.

The use of a wide-body implant and the sequence of steps in the restorative procedures are indicated in Figs. 11.18–11.24.

Conclusions

With immediate implant placement, the four essential conditions for success can be stated as:

- Atraumatic extraction.
- Intact buccal and lingual/palatal plates.
- Absence of purulence/infection.
- Initial implant stability (abutment torque ≥ 30 N.cm).

Clearly, other factors can play an important role in the success or failure of an immediate implant but, in our experience, these four appear to be critical regarding successful placement of an immediate dental implant. However, as discussed in Chapter 15, ensuring absence of mobility in an immediate implant and occlusal overloading following placement can be important determinants in osseointegration, without which successful placement of an implant can be very questionable.

Reference

1. Massa, L. and von Fraunhofer, J.A. (2018). Socket grafting large defects with delayed implant placement. *EC Dent. Sci.* 17 (12): 2207–2212.

12

Full Arch Cases

The global prevalence of complete edentulism is increasing [1] and its effects on patients is of increasing concern. In particular, edentulous patients are limited physically because of difficulties in chewing or speaking clearly as well as suffering psychological and social limitations due to a compromised facial appearance as well as an increased reluctance to smile [2]. Nowadays, the optimal approach to addressing edentulism and its associated problems is the use of endosseous dental implants supporting fixed or removable dental prostheses. In fact, placing two or more implants, with the number of implants placed depending on which jaw is under restoration and the specifics of the case in question, is now the standard of care for restoring an edentulous arch [3–5].

A full arch case is defined as replacing an entire arch with an implant-supported prosthesis. This area of implant dentistry has become increasingly popular due to an overwhelming need and an increased education in the patient population. Implant dentistry has made traditional dentures less desirable. But, unfortunately, the costs associated with implant-retained prostheses can make traditional dentures the only viable option for many patients.

We find that edentulous patients generally dislike almost every aspect of wearing complete dentures (CDs) and many general dentists prefer not to deal with CD patients for many and often varied reasons. Not least of which being that it can often be almost impossible to provide an enduring and completely satisfactory solution for patients in addressing their problems.

These patient and dentist complaints regarding CDs include but are not limited to the factors indicated in Table 12.1.

The ADA Practical Guide to Dental Implants, First Edition. Luigi O. Massa and J. Anthony von Fraunhofer.
© 2021 The American Dental Association. Published 2021 by John Wiley & Sons, Inc.

Table 12.1 Patient/clinician concerns with complete dentures.

Poor retention, notably lower dentures
Esthetics (caved-in facial appearance)
Loss of facial vertical dimension
Masticatory pain
Impaired oral hygiene and malodor
Susceptibility to irritation from food particles trapped beneath the denture
Malocclusion
TMJ problems
Denture staining and wear
Susceptibility to oral thrush/candidiasis
Impaired taste, thermal and texture sensitivity
Ridge resorption
Need for continuous cleaning and sterilization
Stimulation of the gag reflex
Frequent need for retention aids
Awareness of a foreign body in the mouth
Restricted masticatory and incisal efficacy

Of course, many of these issues are inter-related such as poor retention and resorbed ridges following extraction. Likewise, there is commonly a relationship between malocclusion, ridge resorption and temporomandibular joint (TMJ) problems. All of which can contribute to masticatory pain and discomfort.

Poor oral hygiene, denture odor and candida infections can be very common with CDs as are staining and wear of the denture(s) together with poor esthetics. Many of these patient-related problems can be addressed by regular and efficient/effective cleansing of the prosthesis as well as the daily use of anti-bacterial mouthwashes. It is ironic, as mentioned elsewhere in this book, that CD (and removable partial denture [RPD]) wearers must be diligent with regard to both oral and prosthesis hygiene to avoid disease, oral malodor and many other adverse effects associated with wearing prostheses. If such care had been exercised when the patient was dentate, perhaps the need for dentures might have been avoided.

Certain "cons" of CDs, however, cannot be eliminated, notably impairment of taste, lack of hot/cold sensitivity and the psychological impact of a foreign body (or bodies) within the oral cavity. Further, most CD wearers are aware that they cannot exert more than 50% of the masticatory force that was possible when dentate and biting into hard foodstuffs such as apples, corn-on-the-cob and the like usually presents problems for these patients. For these reasons, as evidenced by the plethora of TV commercials regarding the convenience and successes associated with implant dentistry, increasing numbers of patients are seeking to replace CDs by implant-supported prostheses.

Treatment Modalities for the Edentulous Patient

The full arch implant case is the most complex case in dentistry today. It involves many factors including biological, functional (occlusal) and esthetic. For this reason, we will limit our discussion to two types of prostheses: The implant over-denture and the fixed implant bridge.

Implant Overdentures

Implant overdentures are removable appliances which are both implant- and tissue-borne prostheses and utilize an abutment and a denture attachment for the retention. Figure 12.1 shows the pre-operative panoramic radiograph of a terminal dentition and Figure 12.2 shows the placement of implants following extraction and bone healing. The male attachment can be situated within the prosthesis (Fig. 12.3) whereas the female component in this example surmounts an implant within the jawbone.

These appliances solve several major problems with traditional dentures, notably:

* Provide greater masticatory forces (≥50% of that for dentate patients)
* Improved incisal capacity
* Increased retention/no denture adhesives needed

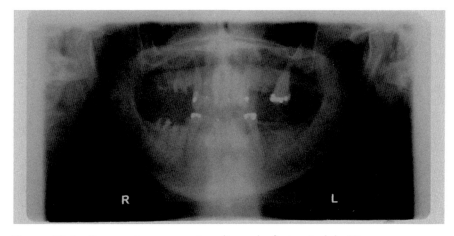

Figure 12.1   Pre-operative panoramic radiograph of a terminal dentition.

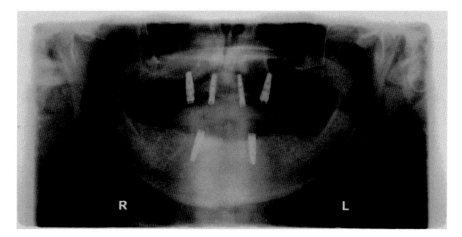

Figure 12.2   Implant placement.

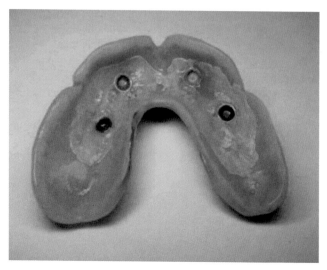

Figure 12.3 Intaglio view of the male attachments within the prosthesis.

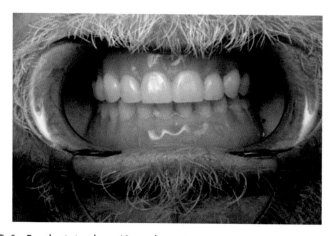

Figure 12.4 Prosthesis in place 48 months post-op.

- Possible elimination of palatal coverage for patients who cannot tolerate the denture due to gag reflex
- Improved taste, thermal and sensory capability if the palatal coverage is eliminated
- Reduced awareness of foreign bodies in the mouth
- Improved occlusion and reduced TMJ problems assuming correct vertical dimension

An implant-supported over-denture can be a wholly satisfactory and viable economic alternative to the traditional CD (Fig.12.4) although there are, of course, some disadvantages to the use of implants to replace multiple missing teeth (Table 12.2). Nevertheless, a great many CD patients and those about to become edentulous opt for implant-supported overdentures to address the problems and issues cited earlier.

Table 12.2   Disadvantages of implants vs traditional CD, bridgework, and RPDs.

Short-term cost is higher than for a traditional CD
Surgery is required
Generally, treatment time is longer – 3–6 months
Regular maintenance is required

Table 12.3   Treatment protocols for providing root implants and implant-supported dentures for both dentate and edentulous patients.

Dentate Patient	Edentulous Patient
1. Initial impressions for immediate denture 2. Evaluate jaw relations 3. Evaluate wax try-in 4. Extraction/alveoplasty, implant placement, delivery of immediate denture (implant placement may be immediate or delayed) 5. Tissue conditioning 6. Final impressions for overdenture with healing abutments in place 7. Evaluate jaw relations 8. Evaluate wax try-in 9. Final delivery/pick-up with attachments	1. Reline of existing dentures 2. Implant placement 3. Final impressions for overdenture with healing abutments in place 4. Evaluate jaw relations 5. Evaluate wax try-in 6. Final delivery/ pick-up of attachments

(a)   (b)

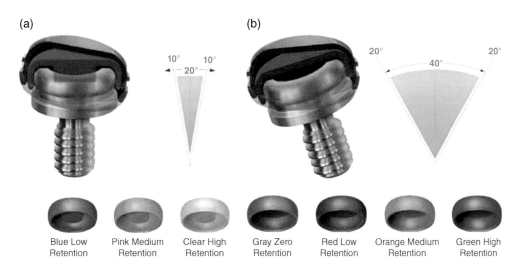

| Blue Low Retention | Pink Medium Retention | Clear High Retention | Gray Zero Retention | Red Low Retention | Orange Medium Retention | Green High Retention |

Figure 12.5   (a) and (b) Male attachments (*Source*: Zest Anchors.).

The treatment protocols for providing root implants and implant-supported dentures for both dentate and edentulous patients are outlined in Table 12.3.

Because both root and implant-supported overdentures have somewhat unique clinical requirements and objectives, specialized attachments have been developed for these particular treatment modalities.

The attachments comprise the male part utilized in the prosthesis, Figs. 12.5a,b, and the female part, which is placed in the jaw or tooth root, Fig. 12.6.

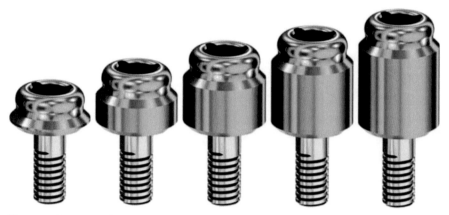

Figure 12.6   Female abutments (*Source*: Zest Anchors.).

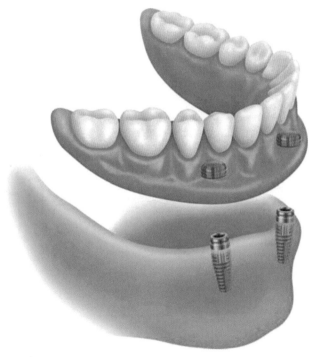

Figure 12.7   Implant-supported overdenture.

The implant-supported denture, Fig. 12.7, is an excellent option for the edentulous or pre-edentulous patient.

Fixed Implant Bridge(S)

While an implant supported overdenture provides satisfactory results to many patients, it is still a removable appliance and many patients hold negative connotations with removable appliances and, in fact, several negative factors nevertheless do exist. Plastics and acrylics have improved greatly but to many patients and dentists, they are inferior to materials such as zirconia. For these reasons, fixed implant full arch restorations are the optimal treatment option in many cases.

Fixed implant bridges are a completely implant-borne prosthesis whereas the implant overdenture is a tissue and implant-borne prosthesis. The fixed implant bridge can be categorized into two main restorations:

* A teeth-only replacement bridge, or
* A teeth and tissue replacement bridge.

A teeth-only replacement bridge is also commonly known as a "crown and bridge restoration" (Figs. 12.8 and 12.9) and follows much of the same criteria of a traditional three-unit bridge that is delivered onto prepared teeth. A teeth and

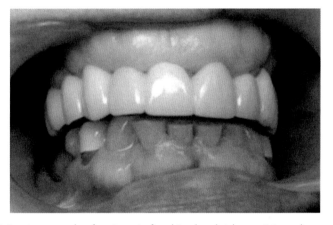

Figure 12.8   An example of a zirconia fixed implant bridge at 24 months.

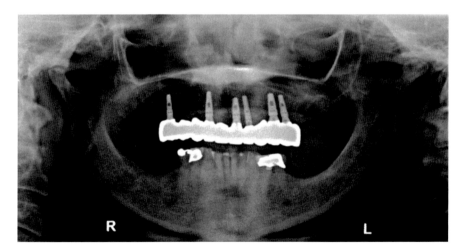

Figure 12.9   Radiograph of the zirconia fixed implant bridge at 24 months.

(a)   (b)

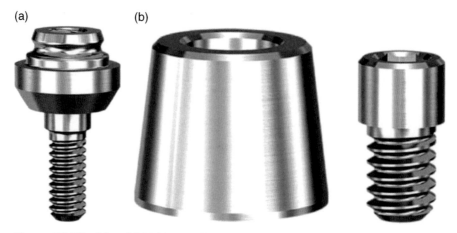

Figure 12.10   (a) and (b) Multi-unit abutment and multiunit cap (*Source*: Implant Direct).

tissue replacement bridge is also more commonly known as a "hybrid restoration" and follows many of the same criteria as a CD.

The advantages of fixed implant bridges are:

a. No need for the patient to remove appliance
b. Function is restored
c. Biocompatible materials like zirconia can be used

The disadvantages of fixed implant bridges are:

i. Cost, generally substantially greater than for overdentures
ii. More intensive to repair
iii. Regular maintenance is required
iv. There can also be a lack of proprioception in an extensive prosthetic case.

The most widely accepted appliance is a *"fixed-detachable"* appliance. A fixed-detachable prosthesis is defined as a prosthesis which is readily retrievable. The most common way this is accomplished is by fabricating a screw-retained prosthesis. Generally, four to six implants are placed in the arch and components are available to allow the prosthesis to draw on these implants. A multi-unit abutment (Fig.12.10) is the most common component used to accomplish this. Multi-unit abutments are also called *screw-receiving abutments* as the appliance is screwed into these abutments.

Material Selection

A widely used approach to providing an implant-supported fixed-detachable prostheses, also known as a fixed CD or hybrid prosthesis, is a titanium bar supporting acrylic resin "gum work" or base and denture teeth [5]. Despite the popularity and wide-spread use of this approach, it has been found that prosthetic (basically biomaterials) complications are far more common than biological ones with this treatment [6, 7]. In particular, the most common biomaterials complication with metal-acrylic hybrid restorations is wear of posterior denture teeth [8].

This problem is now addressed by utilizing monolithic zirconia implant-supported fixed complete dental prostheses [9]. The advantage of using zirconia are its biomechanical properties, notably a fracture toughness of up to 6 MPa·m$^{1/2}$ and an extremely high flexural strength (≤1200 MPa) [10]. These strength characteristics, combined with its esthetic qualities, are the reasons for using zirconia to fabricate monolithic prostheses, especially in situations where there is limited vertical interocclusal space.

A recent retrospective study of full-arch zirconia implant-supported prostheses found less than 1% of fractures in over 2000 cases [9]. Wear of such prostheses is not a clinical concern because zirconia exhibits exceptional wear-resistance [11]. However, in contrast, it has been found that the most common complication associated with monolithic zirconia hybrid restorations was wear of opposing restorations [8, 12–14].

Conclusions

Patients who are edentulous or who will lose their remaining teeth in the near future should be given options to restore their dentition. Many problems exist with traditional dentures – primarily poor retention. Implants can be used to stabilize dentures with the use of abutments or attachments. Implants can also be used to give the patient a fixed alternative. These fixed alternatives are generally screw-retained prostheses that restore the form, function, and esthetics of the natural dentition.

References

1. Douglass, C.W., Shih, A., and Ostry, L. (2002). Will there be a need for complete dentures in the United States in 2020? *J. Prosthet. Dent.* 87: 5–8.
2. Anjum, M.S., Monica, M., Rao, K.Y. et al. (2017). Does tooth loss have an emotional effect? A cross-sectional and comparative study on nondenture wearers and complete denture wearers. *J. Indian Assoc. Public Health Dent.* 15 (3): 247–251.
3. Brånemark, P.I., Adell, R., Breine, U. et al. (1969). Intra-osseous anchorage of dental prostheses. I. Experimental studies. *Scand. J. Plast. Reconstr. Surg.* 3: 81–100.
4. Zarb, G.A. and Zarb, F.L. (1985). Tissue integrated dental prostheses. *Quintessence Int.* 16: 39–42.
5. Sadowsky, S.J. (2007). Treatment considerations for maxillary implant overdentures: a systematic review. *J. Prosthet. Dent.* 97: 340–348.
6. Papaspyridakos, P., Chen, C.J., Chuang, S.K. et al. (2012). A systematic review of biologic and technical complications with fixed implant rehabilitations for edentulous patients. *Int. J. Oral Maxillofac. Implants* 27: 102–110.
7. Dhima, M., Paulusova, V., Lohse, C. et al. (2014). Practice-based evidence from 29-year outcome analysis of management of the edentulous jaw using osseointegrated dental implants. *J. Prosthodont.* 23: 173–181.
8. Box, V.H., Sukotjo, C., Knoernschild, K.L. et al. (2018). Patient-reported and clinical outcomes of implant-supported fixed complete dental prostheses: a comparison of metal-acrylic, milled zirconia, and retrievable crown prostheses. *J. Oral Implantol.* 44: 51–61.

9. Bidra, A.S., Tischler, M., and Patch, C. (2018). Survival of 2039 complete arch fixed implant-supported zirconia prostheses: a retrospective study. *J. Prosthet. Dent.* 119: 220–224.

10. Park, J.H., Park, S., Lee, K. et al. (2014). Antagonist wear of three CAD/CAM anatomic contour zirconia ceramics. *J. Prosthet. Dent.* 111: 20–29.

11. Janyavula, S., Lawson, N., Cakir, D. et al. (2013). The wear of polished and glazed zirconia against enamel. *J. Prosthet. Dent.* 109: 22–29.

12. Maló, P., Araújo Nobre, M.D., Lopes, A., and Rodrigues, R. (2015). Double full-arch versus single full-arch, four implant-supported rehabilitations: a retrospective, 5-year cohort study. *J. Prosthodont.* 24: 263–270.

13. Gonzalez, J. and Triplett, R.G. (2017). Complications and clinical considerations of the implant-retained zirconia complete-arch prosthesis with various opposing dentitions. *Int. J. Oral Maxillofac. Implants* 32: 864–869.

14. Cardelli, P., Manobianco, F.P., Serafini, N. et al. (2016). Full-arch, implant-supported monolithic zirconia rehabilitations: pilot clinical evaluation of wear against natural or composite teeth. *J. Prosthodont.* 25: 629–633.

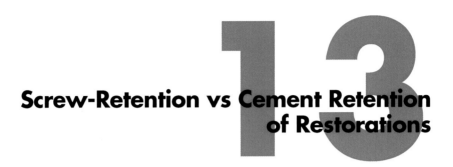

Screw-Retention vs Cement Retention of Restorations

Stability of the connections between the different parts of the overall implant system is a significant factor in the clinical success of the reconstruction. This is especially true for single-tooth restorations, where there is a need for a strong interlock between abutment and implant. The implant-abutment connection stability is influenced by factors such as component fit, machining accuracy, saliva contamination and screw preload.

Attaching the final restoration to the abutment by a screw or dental cement was addressed briefly in Chapters 3, 6, and 11. Which approach is "better" is still a matter of debate. Some clinicians prefer screw-retention and others choose to use a resin-based or adhesive resin "cement" to retain the restoration, Fig. 13.1.

Cement Retention of Restorations

The present international consensus is that cement retention may be recommended for the following situations:

- For short-span prostheses with margins at or above the tissue level
- To enhance esthetics when the screw access passes through the buccal aspect of a restoration
- In cases of malpositioned implants
- To reduce initial treatment costs
- Situations in which access is severely restricted or the patient has limited ability to maximize opening of the jaws.

The ADA Practical Guide to Dental Implants, First Edition. Luigi O. Massa and J. Anthony von Fraunhofer.
© 2021 The American Dental Association. Published 2021 by John Wiley & Sons, Inc.

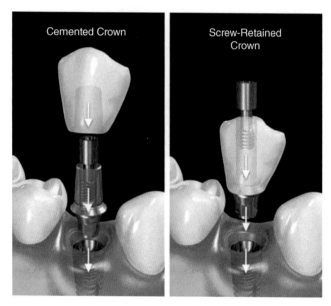

Figure 13.1 Cement and screw-retention of crowns (*Source*: Courtesy of Implant Direct).

Using cement retention will often simplify laboratory fabrication procedures for the restoration. Resorting to cement retention of the restoration to the abutment may be the **only** approach to satisfactorily join restoration and implant, particularly if access to the implant is restricted. Finally, in some instances, there is an esthetic benefit in having intact restorative surfaces, for example, screw access traversing the buccal aspect on an anterior tooth.

However, there can be problems associated with cement-retained restorations, notably if the restoration should fail or need to be replaced. In such cases, removing the cemented restoration from the abutment can present a far greater challenge than simply unscrewing it. Another and important factor regarding cement-retained restorations is that there is always a finite thickness of cement film between restoration and abutment. One consequence of this is that if a viscous cement was used or there is a thick cement film, the restoration may not seat completely down on the abutment. Consequently, there can be a gap between the margins of the restoration and the abutment collar, (Fig. 13.2). Inability to completely seat restorations is well-known in prosthodontics, and the gap at the external line angle can be quite large [1, 2].

The presence of such a gap can result in a multitude of issues, including leaching out of the cement. The latter will permit ingress of fluids and bacteria which may lead to quite significant problems, namely peri-implant bone loss.

It should also be noted that one cause of peri-implantitis is implant-related cement sepsis, which is often a result of excess cement extruding into the peri-implant tissue. Consequences of the latter include increased bleeding on probing, suppuration, and possibly peri-implant attachment loss. Clinical studies indicate that excess cement in the peri-implant tissue may be exacerbated with larger diameter implant fixtures. It appears, however, that the presence of excess cement is often dependent upon the type of cement and, for example, a specialized

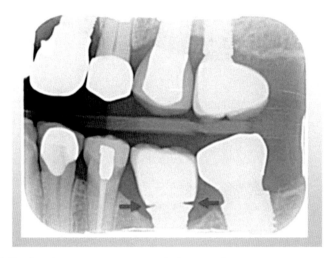

Figure 13.2 Gap between restoration and abutment due to cementation.

methacrylate implant cement favored the development of suppuration and the growth of periodontal pathogens. This subject is discussed again in Chapter 14.

It is of utmost importance that if a cement-retained restoration is indicated, the abutment must be at, or only slightly below, the tissue level (0.5 mm). This will allow for proper removal of any excess cement.

Screw-Retained Restorations

One area of constant concern for implant clinicians is the potential for peri-implantitis associated with cemented crowns and which occasionally leads to implant failure. In order to reduce this risk and eliminate possible complications from cement fixation, many dentists advocate the use of screw-retained crowns and bridges, Fig. 13.3.

Screw retention of restorations may be recommended for the following situations:

- In situations of minimal inter-arch space
- To avoid a cement margin and thus the possibility of cement residue
- When retrievability of the restoration is important or potentially necessary
- In the esthetic zone, to facilitate tissue contouring and conditioning in the transition zone (i.e., developing the emergence profile)

It should be mentioned that to facilitate screw retention, it is recommended that the implant be placed in a prosthetically driven position.

Various mechanisms have been proposed to connect the dental implant abutment to the implant body or fixture and the different systems vary in connection geometry, materials, and overall screw mechanics. Some of these differences were indicated in Chapter 3. It is not uncommon, however, for clinicians to be concerned that the abutment screw can loosen over time. However, the literature [3]

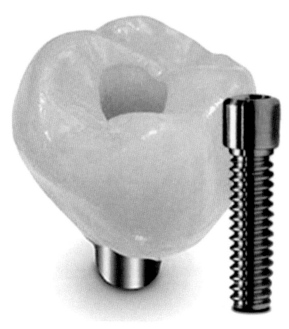

Figure 13.3   Screw-retention of a crown.

indicates that abutment screw loosening is a rare event in single-implant restorations and the survival rate of single-implant restorations after 5.2 years was 98.4% [4]. One reason for this remarkably high success rate is the mechanics involved in attaching the restoration screw to the abutment.

Regardless of the precise screw and abutment design, contaminants such as salivary fluids and blood can seep into the abutment screw hole as well as coat the screw threads during the restoration attachment process. This effect, together with the presence of surface coatings, will change the coefficients of friction for the surfaces being screwed together in the implant complex. Such changes in frictional behavior can affect resistance to screw loosening through their effect on the preload, residual, and removal torque. Recent studies, however, indicate that the amount of removal torque required to loosen the abutment screw was less than the insertion torque at all frictional conditions. On the other hand, decreasing the coefficient of friction at the mating surfaces increases the resistance to screw loosening by its effect on increasing the remaining or residual torque. In other words, if clinicians deliberately contaminate the abutment screw with biologically-compatible lubricants, then removal torque may be increased, reducing the risk of screw loosening. There are also indications that the use of gold-coated screws could also be preferred over non-coated screws because their use would decrease the coefficient of friction at the screw-abutment interface, thereby enhancing resistance to screw loosening by increasing the residual torque.

There is, however, one important issue regarding screw-retained crowns and that is the effect of the screw access hole on the strength of the crown. Screw access holes will disturb the continuity of the occlusal surface and reduce restoration strength, this reduction, depending on the crown material, can be as great as

50%. The lowered restoration strength may result in a susceptibility to fracture in patients with heavy bites, and parafunctional habits such as bruxers.

It should be noted that a problematic implant crown that has been placed with a temporary cement or a low-retention adhesive can be removed and repaired or temporarily replaced with a readily fabricated temporary crown until the permanent replacement is available. In contrast, if problems develop with a screw-retained crown, the latter can be more difficult and expensive to repair or replace, and temporization may present greater difficulties than with a cemented crown. This dichotomy has led to the development of hybridized screw-retained crowns (screw-mentable) with prefabricated, lab-placed screw access holes in a zirconia or lithium silicate/disilicate material that are cemented to the implant fixture (Ti-base), but which may be cleaned extra-orally. The underlying concept is that such hybrids may reduce the risk of future complications with pure screw-retained or cemented crowns.

Despite this seeming controversy between the two approaches to crown-implant retention, it appears from clinical reports that the success rates of screw- and cement-retained restorations are equivalent in the anterior maxillae [5]. The overall implant survival rate was 96.4% and there was no statistically significant difference in survival between the screw- and cement-retained groups. Further, the majority of clinician- and patient-assessed outcomes were similar. The results of this study indicate that for the majority of clinician- and patient-assessed success parameters, screw and cement-retained restorations are equivalent in the anterior maxilla.

Consequently, the subject of restoration selection for screw retention is discussed in some detail in Chapter 14.

Conclusions

The main two restorative options for the implant prosthesis are the screw-retained prosthesis and cement-retained prosthesis. The screw-retained prosthesis is a "one-piece" prosthesis that is directly torqued to the implant through an access hole in the restoration. Generally, the access hole is filled in with a material to protect the screw (Teflon tape, cotton pellet, or polyvinyl siloxane [PVS]) and composite. The major benefits of the screw-retained prosthesis are ease of retrievability and avoiding a cement margin. Cement residue in the sulcus of the implant is known to cause peri-mucositis and peri-implantitis. The cement-retained prosthesis is a two-piece prosthesis consisting of an abutment and the restoration. The abutment is torqued to the implant and then the restoration is cemented to the abutment. Generally, the screw is protected by placing Teflon tape, a cotton pellet, or PVS in the abutment prior to cementation. The main benefit of the cement-retained prosthesis is keeping the restorative material intact.

References

1. McLean, J.W. and von Fraunhofer, J.A. (1971). The estimation of cement film thickness by an *in vivo;* technique. *Br. Dent. J.* 131: 107–111.
2. Dimashkieh, M.R., Davies, E.H., and von Fraunhofer, J.A. (1974). Measurement of the cement film thickness beneath full crown restorations. *Br. Dent. J.* 137: 281–284.

3. Theoharidou, A., Petridis, H.P., Tzannas, K., and Garefis, P. (2007). Abutment screw loosening in single-implant restorations: a systematic review. *Int. J. Oral Maxillofac. Implants* 23 (4): 681–690.

4. Tey, V.H.S., Phillips, R., and Tan, K. (2017). Five-year retrospective study on success, survival and incidence of complications of single crowns supported by dental implants. *Clin. Oral Implants Res.* 28 (5): 620–625.

5. Sherif, S., Susarla, S.M., Hwang, J.W. et al. (2011). Clinician- and patient-reported long-term evaluation of screw- and cement-retained implant restorations: a 5-year prospective study. *Clin. Oral Investig.* 15 (6): 993–999.

14 Restoring Dental Implants

Computer-aided design/computer-aided manufacturing (CAD-CAM) technology was originally developed and commercialized for industrial manufacturing but is of growing importance within dentistry. In fact, it has virtually revolutionized the fabrication of crowns and bridgework and has become the preferred method of making crowns and fixed partial dentures. In contrast to conventional dentistry, with an in-house CAD/CAM system, the dentist typically can fabricate and lute a prosthesis the same day.

Continuing developments in computer-based dental technologies have provided the dental profession with new opportunities for improved clinical workflow and, as indicated above, facilitated manufacturing of dental restorations. Over the last decade or so, CAD/CAM of dental restorations became an established fabrication process, especially for all-ceramic restorations. With the more recent introduction of intraoral scanning systems, digital techniques are now capable of replacing conventional treatment workflow. Numerous clinical trials have demonstrated that single-tooth restorations fabricated in a completely digitized workflow have a clinical fit that is equal to, or better than, conventionally fabricated restorations. Further, when compared with conventional impressions, digital impressions can be more time-efficient and improve the treatment comfort for patients, and clinicians.

In addition to ongoing improvements in digital technologies, new restorative materials that are optimized for CAD/CAM processing have led to further advances and optimization of digital workflows. Biomaterials research in recent years has focused on the development of materials that offer a combination of adequate translucency, improved mechanical strength, and optimized timesaving machining.

The ADA Practical Guide to Dental Implants, First Edition. Luigi O. Massa and J. Anthony von Fraunhofer.
© 2021 The American Dental Association. Published 2021 by John Wiley & Sons, Inc.

CAD/CAM Dentistry

Although most dentists may be familiar to some degree with CAD/CAM dentistry, a brief discussion might be useful here. This is because the predominant trend in dental implantology is to take maximum advantage of digital technology in almost every aspect of the process other than the physical surgical implant placement.

There are numerous systems for digital restoration processing and although specific details vary with each system, all rely upon comparable basics underlying their operation and all CAD/CAM systems contain three components:

- Digital scanner or imaging system
- Software to process the scanned image into data that allows fabrication of the prosthesis
- Hardware that fabricates the prosthesis from the data.

The overall process starts from a three-dimensional (3D) image used by computer software to design the restoration. Imaging systems can now record images of the adjacent and opposing dentition as well as bite registration data. After the information is uploaded into the computer, a data file is assembled which, together with the computer's internal library of tooth shapes, is used to design the restoration.

After the implant and the healing cap are placed and the operative area has healed to the point that there is adequate osseointegration of the implant body, an image or scan is taken of the implant (or implants) and the adjacent/abutment teeth utilizing an intra-oral scanner (Fig. 14.1). Some clinicians, however, will scan the operative area at the time of implant placement to allow for restorative planning.

This image or digital impression is digitized by the recording software in the scanner and the data fed into a computer. Proprietary software then creates a virtual restoration, i.e., a prosthesis that replaces the missing dentition (Fig. 14.2). In technological terms, this process is termed *reverse engineering* and constitutes the CAD part of the overall operation. The software transmits this virtual data to a milling machine where the prosthesis is machined out of a solid (monolithic) block of ceramic or composite resin (Fig. 14.3). The latter process is the CAM part of the operation. Stains and glazes can be fired onto the surfaces of the milled ceramic crown or bridge to correct the otherwise monochromatic appearance of the restoration, Figure 14.4. The restoration is then adjusted in the patient's mouth and cemented or screwed in place.

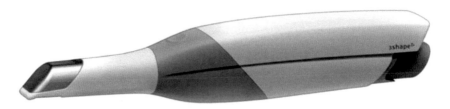

Figure 14.1 Intra-oral scanner.

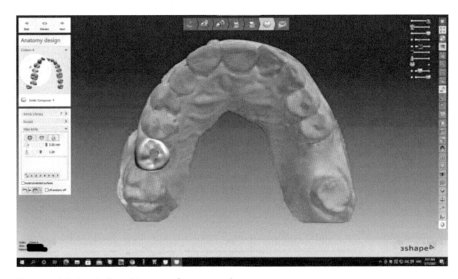

Figure 14.2   A digital image of a scanned cast.

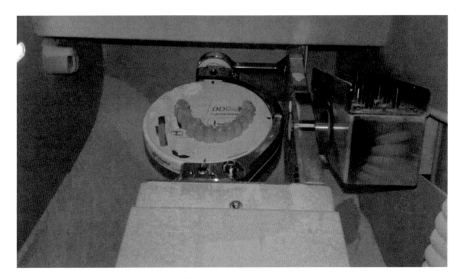

Figure 14.3   A completed CAD/CAM fabricated restoration.

The CAD/CAM systems can either be used chair-side with the restoration fabricating hardware in an adjoining laboratory or the digital data is fed to a remote production center.

Typically, CAD/CAM dental restorations for implants are milled from solid (monolithic) blocks of ceramic or composite resin closely matching the basic shade of the restored tooth or adjacent teeth. Metal alloys may also be milled or digitally produced, often for the posterior teeth in patients with heavy bites and/ or bruxers. The choice of restorative material is discussed below.

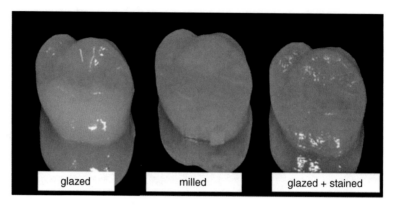

Figure 14.4   Finishing and characterization of a CAD-CAM ceramic restoration (*Source:* Courtesy of Sirona Dental Inc., Charlotte, NC).

It should be mentioned that additive manufacturing (once known as rapid prototyping) has now entered CAD/CAM dentistry. At first, additive manufacturing, also known as *3D printing*, was almost an experimental laboratory approach to fabricating dental restorations but now there is increasing interest in the scope of its applicability in dentistry. The underlying concept of additive manufacturing is in complete contrast to the *subtractive manufacturing* process of milling the object (prosthesis) from a solid block.

The term *3D printing* is commonly applied to all types of additive manufacturing, but this term should refer only to fabricating objects through the deposition of a material using printer technology such as a printer head or precision spray nozzle. In fact, "additive manufacturing" strictly refers to the construction of objects from 3D data, usually layer-by-layer until fabrication is complete. The three most common additive manufacturing methods are Selective Laser Sintering (SLS), Direct Metal Laser Sintering (DMLS) and Selective Laser Melting (SLM). SLS and DMLS are basically the same process in that the applied laser beam coalesces the particles in the deposited material through partial fusion but without achieving a full melt. When this sintering methodology is used for non-metallic materials, it is commonly referred to as SLS whereas DMLS is the term used for processing metallic particles. In contrast, with SLM technology, the metal particles are fully melted and then cooled to consolidate the constructed object. Although the two processes are somewhat similar, the major difference is that with SLM, the processed objects do not have the porosity found with DMLS because the complete melting/cooling cycle of the deposited particles ensures greater solidity and density of the fabricated object.

Advantages and Drawbacks of CAD/CAM Technology

Many commercial CAD/CAM systems are available, including the CEREC (CERamic REConstruction), Planmeca, E4D, 3Shape Dental and Cera systems. Examples of chair-side and laboratory CAD-CAM systems are shown in Figs. 14.5 and 14.6. In addition to the increasing variety of CAD/CAM systems available, continuing technological advances include increasingly versatile software, direct

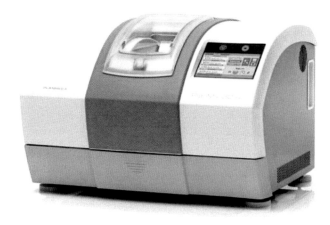

Figure 14.5 A CAD CAM chairside system (*Source:* Courtesy of E4D).

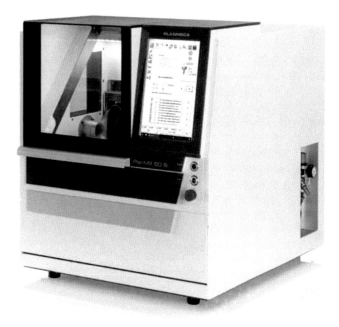

Figure 14.6 A CAD-CAM laboratory system (*Source*: Courtesy of Planmeca).

digital recording of the dentition and CAM units with greater speed and accuracy in milling operations.

Modern dental CAD/CAM technologies based on integrated implantology software enable the dentist to plan the implant treatment and implement the trephining precisely using a surgical guide (Fig. 14.7). Combining CAD/CAM software with 3D-imaging data encourages greater safety and helps prevent problems arising from any intraoperative mistakes.

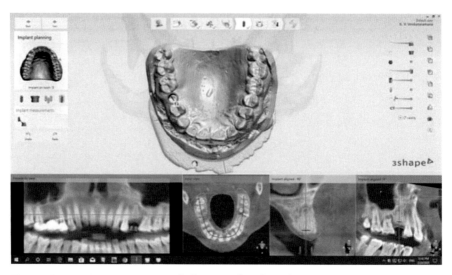

Figure 14.7   Computer-generated planning of implant placement.

Ideally, the CAD/CAM restoration should fit perfectly but CAD/CAM restorations may often require some adjustment to ensure an exact fit with the correct occlusion, particularly with regard to abutment teeth and implant abutments as well as opposing dentition. Fit accuracy can vary with the CAD/CAD system utilized and from user to user, with some systems attaining higher standards of accuracy than others and greater accuracy with more experienced operators.

In general, milling all ceramic restorations from a monolithic block and layering with "enamel" ceramics enables better blending with the surrounding dentition for an esthetic outcome and, ideally, the restored implant will have an anatomically and functionally perfect restoration. CAD/CAM has improved the consistency of dental prostheses and standardized the production process. It has increased laboratory and practice productivity while providing the dentist with an opportunity to work with new materials with a high level of accuracy. Further, digital dentistry enables the dentist to send electronic impressions to the lab so that restorations are milled from a block of ceramic, and these restorations will have fewer flaws and are produced in minutes rather than hours (Fig. 14.8). However, CAD/CAM requires a large initial financial outlay and occlusal detail may often require manual amendment to achieve optimum results. Further, the dentist's technique and operative approach may need to be adapted to the demands of CAD/CAM and milling technology. Typically, this includes correct tooth (abutment) preparations with a continuous preparation margin, typically in the form of a chamfer so that it is recognizable by the scanner. Further, shoulder-less preparations and parallel walls should be avoided as well as preparations having rounded incisor and occlusal edges to avoid stress concentrations.

It must be stressed that there is a learning curve with CAD/CAM technology so that "one-visit" dentistry may not always be possible at first, particularly if multiple post-fabrication adjustments are necessary. Modifying the computer-generated restoration design (the CAD phase of the operation) to achieve optimal margins

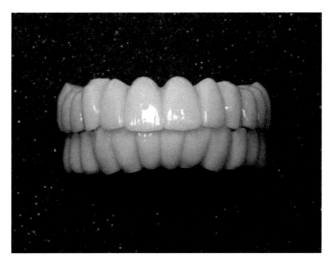

Figure 14.8   Completed CAD/CAM generated full-arch restoration.

and avoid brittle knife edges with ceramic restorations requires practice, experience, and skill.

There are many advantages to using digital restorations for implants, notably significantly faster delivery of the restoration compared to traditional laboratory-fabricated restorations and potentially fewer patient visits. Further, with monolithic ceramic restorations, minor adjustments are relatively easy to make without the need for reglazing or heat treatment and/or recasting of metal crowns and bridgeworks. It is also possible to refine margins, contacts, and so forth on the CAD pattern before the finished data file is transmitted to the CAM unit for processing.

However, depending upon the system used and the particular case, digital restorations may be approximations rather than exact matches to the patient's dentition and an accurate bite cannot always be guaranteed. As a result, esthetics may be compromised and there is often a risk of an unbalanced occlusion. These effects arise because the technology for CAD-CAM restorative procedures cannot always guarantee good marginal fit and, unfortunately, the margins of ceramic and resin restorations cannot be swaged like gold crowns. However, it must be stated that advances in dental CAD/CAM technology are occurring on an almost daily basis due to software updates and improvements, more comprehensive data banks and improved milling technology within CAM units.

Restorative Materials

Although implants may be restored with cast and metal-ceramic (porcelain-fused-to-metal or PFM) crowns and prostheses, most digital implant restorations are fabricated from high-strength ceramics today. In addition, high-strength composite materials based on restorative resins have been developed specifically for CAD-CAM applications.

Depending on the selected restorative material, however, CAD/CAM-generated restorations can have esthetic limitations, often depending on whether they were created at the dental practice or outsourced to a remote dental laboratory. Nevertheless, contingent on the requirements of the dentist and/or the skill of the technician, CAD/CAM restorations can be layered to give a deeper more natural look, improving esthetics and avoiding a monochromatic appearance.

There are also different radiological ramifications associated with each restorative material. If the CAD/CAM restorative material is zirconia, then the restoration will be radio-opaque, comparable to metal restorations. However, alumina, lithium disilicate and some composite resin materials are radio-lucent, a property that enables the dentist to track potential carious attack on the natural dentition.

Many ceramic digital restorations have high strength, natural translucency and fluorescence combined, usually, with good fit. Further, with some materials such as leucite-reinforced glass–ceramics, restorations can be polished and characterized, (Fig. 14.3). Ceramic restorations also have the major advantage of outstanding chemical resistance and may suffer less from certain problems such as plaque build-up and staining found with other materials. On the other hand, some materials do not possess high flexural strength or fracture toughness and they can cause wear of opposing dentition, as discussed below. It should be mentioned that because CAD/CAM restorations are machined from monolithic material, they are generally stronger than those that are incrementally constructed, e.g., porcelain restorations and multi-layered composites.

As mentioned above, implant crowns in the past were primarily made from PFMs but the modern trend is to use more esthetic all-ceramic crowns made from lithium disilicate or zirconia,[a] with lithium disilicate being preferred in esthetically critical cases. However, little is known about the long-term performance of this material as an implant crown with a screw access hole.

Zirconia-based crowns and prostheses have been used as an alternative to PFM restorations because they are metal-free and have a white color. In fact, zirconia-based restorations are the favored treatment for extensively compromised teeth because of the material's biocompatibility and excellent mechanical properties. On the other hand, because of the material's opacity, zirconia copings often must be veneered with porcelain to improve esthetics but this, unfortunately, results in a bi-layer restoration. Cohesive fracture within the veneering porcelain is one of the most common clinical failures found in veneered zirconia restorations but this problem is averted by CAD/CAM manufacture of zirconia monolithic crowns. Not only can the prostheses be milled in anatomical contour with different levels of translucency, it is possible to improve the esthetics of monolithic restorations by using some staining techniques. As discussed below, monolithic zirconia crowns seem to cause more wear clinically to the opposing enamel than human enamel itself and even other restorative materials and this problem is exacerbated when post-installation occlusal adjustments are required. This is because occlusal adjustments with a diamond bur significantly increases surface roughness of the zirconia which, in turn, increases wear of both the agonist and antagonist surface. Further, inadequate polishing of the zirconia occlusal surface will result in densely distributed cracks throughout that surface which may compromise mechanical properties. This issue is theoretically a problem not just for zirconia but with all glass–ceramics.

CAD-CAM composite resins possess high flexural strength and fracture toughness and their wear characteristics are comparable to those of enamel, obviating damage to opposing dentition. They are easier to finish and polish than ceramics and can be easily characterized using light-cured composite stains. They also have the advantage that restorations can be repaired in the mouth. Further, because composite restorations have a resin matrix, it is relatively easy for the interior (fitting) surfaces to be treated to facilitate bonding. In contrast, ceramic restorations may require hydrofluoric acid etching and silane treatment prior to adhesive bonding. On the other hand, as with all resin-based restorations, they can be subject to staining and wear in use.

Cement retention compared to screw retention of implant restorations was discussed in Chapter 13, but it should be mentioned here that digital restorations are usually luted with dual-cure adhesives although if sufficiently translucent, light-cured adhesives can be used. Light-cured glass ionomer cements (GICs) and resin-modified glass ionomers (RMGIs) are not recommended for all ceramic restorations because hygroscopic expansion can cause fracture over time.

Studies indicate that, depending on the impression technique and the selected restorative material [1, 2], the marginal gap with digital restorations is typically 60–150 µm, i.e., comparable to those with conventional (cast) restorations [3, 4]. If the luting material can be leached out or worn away, particularly with wide or open margins. With restored implants, the frequency of undetected excess cement depends essentially on the type of cement used. Cements that tend to leave more undetected excess such as methacrylate cements have a higher prevalence of peri-implant inflammation and cause more severe peri-implant bone loss compared to a zinc oxide-eugenol cement. Interestingly, it has been found that there is a significantly greater amount of excess cement in the peri-implant tissue with larger diameter implants.

It is also possible that when a precious or semi-precious metal crown has been cemented to a titanium implant, galvanic corrosion can occur, leading to bone necrosis and implant failure. It should be stated, however, that galvanic corrosion at a mixed metal restoration-abutment junction can also occur with screw-retained prostheses.

Wear and Abrasion

Wear of restorations is a complex phenomenon that can be influenced by several factors including the material's microstructure, environmental effects and patient behavior and characteristics. In general, it is accepted that large differences in surface hardness can be a contributing factor to abrasion and wear. On the other hand, it has been found from studies on veneering porcelain that wear had no direct relation with its hardness, but was more a result of its composition and the particle size and distribution of crystals. In fact, there does appear to be a correlation between surface roughness and wear, with abrasivity being a major contributor to wear when the agonist (or antagonist) has a crystal size less than 5 µm. Research studies indicate wear of alumina surfaces caused by lithium disilicate and zirconia is reduced when the surfaces were polished rather than glazed.

Normally, wear leads to loss of the original anatomy and alteration of the vertical dimension of restorations which, in turn, can result in malocclusion. This may cause physiological and pathological disorders as well as esthetically compromise the restoration. Problems associated with wear-exacerbated malocclusions as well as parafunctional habits and bruxing can lead to loosening of implants, especially in the case of single units.

In the past, there have been various studies that looked at the wear of prosthetic, notably denture, teeth against different antagonists and, generally, unfilled cross-linked polymethyl methacrylate resins exhibited less wear than filled composite resins. This almost counter-intuitive finding suggests that the dentist's decision to prescribe artificial teeth and restorative materials for prostheses should be based on considerations of functionality and esthetics, together with the cost of the material.

A widely used material for CAD/CAM restorations is lithium disilicate, a glass–ceramic material similar to but with a far greater strength than porcelain. Lithium disilicate materials are commonly used to fabricate restorations because of their durability, translucency, and close resemblance to the color of natural teeth. Although lithium disilicate is brittle with low elasticity, it has greater fatigue resistance than feldspathic porcelain and, in clinical use, its mechanical properties are far more predictable when used with at least a 1.5 mm thickness for occlusal surfaces.

However, placing a screw access hole in lithium disilicate crowns results in a significant decrease in load-bearing strength and some suggest that the material should not be used for screw-retained restorations. On the other hand, other studies have found no significant difference in the clinical behavior of screw-retained, cemented, or hybridized screw-retained restorations. The consensus appears to be that whereas lithium disilicate is weakened by a central fossa hole, as indicated by early fractures along the central groove, they are still indicated in areas of minimal loading. Despite cement-retained implant crowns being less expensive, seating passively and are easier to work with, the use of screw-retained implant crowns eliminates possible cement-related complications and permits retrievability should screw loosening occur. Interestingly, the majority of clinician- and patient-assessed success parameters indicate that screw- and cement-retained restorations have comparable clinical performance on implants in the anterior maxilla.

Studies of the clinical performance of ceramic single crowns over 5- and 10-year periods support their application in all areas of the mouth. However, with layered ceramic posterior crowns, most fractures of the core occur early in the lifetime of the restoration and monolithic ceramic systems are probably advisable for posterior crowns. Interestingly, research indicates that tooth-supported crowns had a slightly lower or comparable success rate than implant-supported crowns [5, 6] whereas fixed dental lithium disilicate glass–ceramic framework prostheses (FPDs) were found to have 5- and 10-year survival and success rates that were similar to those of conventional metal-ceramic FPDs [7]. Further, it was noted that neither the cementation mode nor positioning of the restoration impacted restoration survival. The consensus is that lithium disilicate is a reliable material for fabricating restorations, especially for the single-unit restoration. Zirconia-based single crowns with a sintered veneering cap showed promising clinical results on both tooth and implant abutments although the dental implants were more prone to complications. Consequently, high-strength ceramic with a sintered veneering cap can be recommended for both tooth- and implant-supported single crowns in molar regions [8].

In situations where prosthetic crowns are required to have greater strength, the material of choice has been zirconia. Zirconia, however, has esthetic limitations and studies have shown that well-polished monolithic zirconia caused similar or more agonist enamel wear than natural enamel, but this wear was less than that with metal-ceramic restorations. Nevertheless, the high hardness and wear resistance of zirconia may adversely affect opposing natural dentition and other indirect restorative materials, especially when the restoration's surface is not perfectly smooth. As previously stated, monolithic zirconia crowns seem to cause more wear to the opposing enamel than human enamel itself.

In order to address these issues, a new group of machinable ceramics has recently been introduced for CAD/CAM techniques. These high-strength ceramics include zirconia-reinforced lithium silicates (ZLS) such as Celtra Duo and Suprinity with superior esthetics. The reinforcement is achieved through the addition of 8–10 wt.% of zirconium oxide (ZrO_2) to the glass–ceramic. These materials have comparable physical properties to lithium disilicate and strengths some 3X greater than traditional leucite-reinforced glass-ceramics. Further, the presence of ZrO_2 results in a more homogeneous structure to the ceramic. Whether there are differences in wear susceptibility between lithium disilicate and ZLS are unknown currently.

Conclusions

Today, most fixed restorations are fabricated utilizing CAD/CAM technology. The process digitizes a standard impression, a stone cast, or the implant itself. Thereafter, the restoration is designed using a specialized software. The design is then sent to a mill which machines the restoration out of the material of choice. The two most common materials utilized for implant restorations today are zirconia and lithium disilicate. Materials used in CAD/CAM technology for dental restorations have many pros and cons to consider and are rapidly evolving.

References

1. Abdel-Azim, T., Rogers, K., Elathamna, E. et al. (2015). Comparison of the marginal fit of lithium disilicate crowns fabricated with CAD/CAM technology by using conventional impressions and two intraoral digital scanners. *J. Prosthet. Dent.* 114 (4): 554–559.
2. Ng, J., Ruse, D., and Wyatt, C. (2014). A comparison of the marginal fit of crowns fabricated with digital and conventional methods. *Journal of Prosthetic Dentistry* 112 (3): 555–560.
3. McLean, J.W. and von Fraunhofer, J.A. (1971). The estimation of cement film thickness by an *in vivo* technique. *Br. Dent. J.* 131: 107–111.
4. Dimashkieh, M.R., Davies, E.H., and von Fraunhofer, J.A. (1974). Measurement of the cement film thickness beneath full crown restorations. *Br. Dent. J.* 137: 281–284.
5. Salinas, T.J. and Eckert, S.E. (2007). In patients requiring single-tooth replacement, what are the outcomes of implant- as compared to tooth-supported restorations? *Int. J. Oral Maxillofac. Implants* 22 (7): 71–107.

6. Pjetursson, B.E., Brägger, U., Niklaus, P. et al. (2007). Comparison of survival and complication rates of tooth-supported fixed dental prostheses (FDPs) and implant-supported FDPs and single crowns (SCs). *Clin. Oral Implants Res.* 18 (3): 97–113.
7. Kern, M., Sasse, M., and Wolfart, S. (2012). Ten-year outcome of three-unit fixed dental prostheses made from monolithic lithium disilicate ceramic. *J. Am. Dent. Assoc.* 143 (3): 234–240.
8. Cantner, F., Cacaci, C., Mücke, T. et al. (2019). Clinical performance of tooth- or implant-supported veneered zirconia single crowns: 42-month results. *Clin. Oral Investig.* 23: 4301–4309.

Note

a Yttria-partially stabilized tetragonal zirconia polycrystal (Y-TZP) is frequently referred to as *zirconia*.

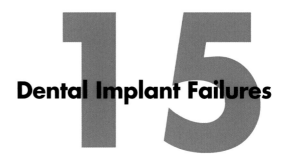

Dental Implant Failures

The literature on potential failures of dental implants tends to be somewhat conflicting, if not confusing. The overall success rate of dental implants is about 95% although some authorities claim that it is higher (i.e., about 98%) whereas others suggest that it might **only** be 93%. Regardless of the precise success-to-failure ratio, dental implants are still one of the most successful procedures a general dentist can perform and, as indicated in Chapter 16, one of the most profitable.

Recognizing a Failing Implant

When there has been inadequate and incomplete osseointegration, the predominant indicator is mobility of the implant. Initially, this mobility may only be detectable by a dentist or hygienist but as failure progresses, the initial limited mobility will progress to movement of the prosthetic crown on mastication and even on talking. Other indications of the lack/loss of osseointegration and potential implant failure may include pain, swelling, or infection although in the long term, once there is significant loss of bone around the implant fixture, progressive evulsion and failure occur.

Despite the incredible success of dental implantology, failures still occur and at a rate of 8.16% in the maxilla and 4.93% in the mandible, regardless of the majority of risk factors [1, 2]. Many factors may be involved in such failures, but these data suggest that, for the average dentist performing 100 implant procedures per year, between 2 and 10 failures will occur on an annual basis. These failures follow what is known as a *stochastic* variation, namely that they are randomly determined and/or distributed. In other words, implant failures occur in a random pattern which may be analyzed statistically but they cannot be predicted precisely,

The ADA Practical Guide to Dental Implants, First Edition. Luigi O. Massa and J. Anthony von Fraunhofer.
© 2021 The American Dental Association. Published 2021 by John Wiley & Sons, Inc.

and they will occur "sporadically." If an implant is placed in a compromised site it is much easier to find a "cause and effect" which may lead to implant failure. Some of these "cause and effects" include poor bone quality, low or no initial stability of the implant, and presence of infection or granulation tissue.

Risk Factors for a Failed Dental Implant

There are many reports in the literature regarding the statistically significant factors that affect implant survival, but the data are not clear-cut. Certain factors may impact the success or failure of implants in both the short-term, i.e., failure within 12 months of surgery, implant placement and restoration – what are known as *early implant failures,* and those occurring long-term, i.e., after 12+ months. The term *early implant failure* also applies to implants that failed prior to restoration and loading.

Broadly speaking, implant failure risks fall into two broad categories: intrinsic and extrinsic.

Intrinsic failures include the following:

- Failure of the implant system or any of its components
- Poor, inadequate, or incomplete osseointegration following placement
- Presence of infection or periodontal disease
- Poor bone quality at the implant site
- Nonideal osteotomy or insertion procedures
- Presence of diabetes mellitus or osteoporotic bone
- Galvanic corrosion between the implant and restorations
- Incorrect or improper selection of the implant

Thus, whereas patient age and gender, body mass index (BMI) may not significantly affect implant survival, success factors such as periodontal disease, smoking and systemic disease can impact implant survival [1–5].

Extrinsic failures are those arising from external influences, including:

- Excessive loading on the implant or the attached prosthesis
- Poor positioning of the implant
- Bruxism
- Malocclusion
- Medications
- Chemotherapy
- Steroids use

Some implant failures may be operator-related, others are ascribable to inherent (intrinsic) issues related to the patient, the quality of bone at the implant site and finally, but relatively rarely, some are due to failure of a component of the implant system.

Overall, it appears that the most reported conditions contributing to implant failure are:

- Non-osseous integration and fibrous encapsulation
- Peri-mucositis

- Peri-implantitis
- Certain prescription medications
- Hardware failure
- Periodontal disease [5]

For clarity in this context, *peri*-implant *mucositis* is gingival inflammation found only around the soft tissues of the dental implant but with no loss of marginal bone beyond normal resorption. Although *peri*-implant *mucositis* may be successfully treated and is reversible if caught early, if untreated, it is a precursor to *peri*-implantitis with its eventual bone destruction and loss of the implant.

In contrast, oral mucositis (OM) is an inflammatory, erosive and/or ulcerative process within the mouth, usually caused by radiation or chemotherapy. OM is often accompanied by severe pain and difficulty in eating, and can severely impact a person's quality of life, nutritional intake, and continuing treatment for cancer.

Operator Experience

It is interesting that, in contrast to the quite extensive data available on patient-related and implant component factors in early implant failures, there is relatively little reported information available on the surgeon's role in early implant failures. However, in relative terms, dentists that place more implants in sites with poor bone quality have a greater overall percentage of early implant failures. Placing implants in compromised sites can sometimes be due to lack of experience but may not always be avoidable. This is almost predictable since bone quality at the implant site is one determining factor in the success or failure of the implant.

One major study [6] has addressed this operator issue by analyzing implant failures that occurred after a total of 11 074 implant operations were performed at a specialist clinic over a period of 28 years. The study evaluated the results for 8808 individual patients treated by 23 different dentists, 21 of whom were specialists in oral surgery or periodontology. Of these large number of operations, early implant failures were found for only 616 operations (5.6%). Interestingly, most of these failures occurred with edentulous upper jaws. It was also found that there were statistically significant differences between male and female surgeons, implants placed in maxillae vs mandibles and the nature of the implant surface. The study indicated that although early failure rates decreased when implant bodies with a moderately roughened surface were placed, the relationship between failure rates and surgeons stayed the same although it is likely that case selection and operator experience contributed to the observed data.

Hardware Failure

There is little data available on relative success/failure rates for different types of implants or those from different manufacturers. It appears overall, however, that implant height (i.e., body length), implant type (cylindrical or tapered) and one-stage or two-stage placement has no statistically significant effect on success or failure although many studies directed at these effects were not well controlled. Nevertheless, the literature indicates that modern implants with tapered bodies and roughened surfaces exhibit higher success rates than the early smooth surface implant bodies.

It should be mentioned here that mini-mplants, i.e., those with narrower diameters and platforms are recommended for very limited sites, i.e., those with minimal access or close spacing between remaining teeth. The corollary to this is that the mass of implant osseointegrated with bone is less than that with a conventional implant. Due to these factors, mini-implants should be used with caution.

Failure of implant hardware is unusual, if not comparatively rare. An interesting example is the following. An implant was restored using a custom milled Ti base/zirconia restoration, (Fig. 15.1).

The patient complained that the restoration appeared to be loose and the dentist simply torqued it back in place. When the restoration crown loosened again, clinical examination indicated that the "hex" of the titanium implant body had fractured off and the anti-rotation protection was lost, (Fig. 15.2a,b).

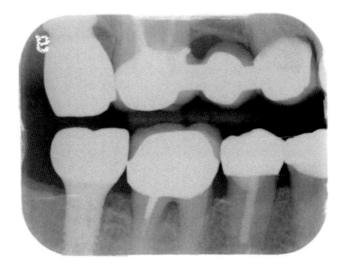

Figure 15.1   Radiograph of a restored Atlantis Ti-base implant restoration.

(a)   (b)

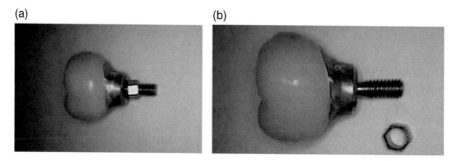

Figure 15.2 (a) Fractured hexagonal internal connection. (b) Restoration showing fractured hexagonal internal connection.

In this particular case, the implant was solidly osseointegrated so that it was possible to take an impression, replace the abutment and provide a restoration to the final torque resistance without difficulty.

This situation is actually comparatively rare and appears to only occur with patients who are heavy bruxers. It is possible that such failures may be preventable by prescribing a bite guard so that undue occlusal forces on the implant and restoration are avoided.

Effects of Medications

It is now accepted, and confirmed by various clinical studies, that certain medications adversely affect the success of dental implants. These predominantly appear to be antidepressants and bisphosphonates.

Antidepressants

According to the Centers for Disease Control and Prevention (CDC), at least 1 in 10 Americans over the age of 12 use antidepressants., which are now the second most prescribed type of drug in the U.S. The rate of antidepressant use is increasing, having risen by 400% between the periods 1988–1994 and 2005–2008 [7].

Clinical studies indicate that antidepressants such as serotonin reuptake inhibitors (SSRIs) are likely to double the failure rates of dental implants because of their effects on bone metabolism. In particular, SSRIs appear to reduce bone formation, increase osteoclast differentiation and inhibit osteoblast proliferation, all of which potentially contribute to osteoporosis [8]. Failure rates may also be higher for non-SSRI antidepressants [9].

Bisphosphonates

Bisphosphonate (BP) therapy is commonly used for the treatment of osteoporosis for cancer, Paget's disease and various other conditions [10]. The route of bisphosphonate administration affects the skeletal uptake in that intravenous (IV) bisphosphonates are completely bioavailable, oral bisphosphonates are poorly absorbed and have less than 1% bioavailability. Whereas the clinical data indicate that patients who have received IV bisphosphonates are at high risk for osteonecrosis in the mandible and maxilla, the situation for patients who have taken oral bisphosphonates is less clear. Although the data on the association between oral bisphosphonates, osteonecrosis, and dental implant failure is limited, there is increasing evidence that long-term oral therapy may lead to Bisphosphonate Related Osteonecrosis of the Jaws (BRONJ). However, because of the growing number of osteonecrosis cases in the jaws associated with various antiresorptive and antiangiogenic therapies, the American Association of Oral and Maxillofacial Surgeons (AAOMS) in 2014 suggested a nomenclature change from BRONJ to Medication Related Osteonecrosis of the Jaw or MRONJ [11].

A systematic review of the literature performed in 2016 [12] indicated that 8.49% of patients with history of bisphosphonate use experienced implant loss and 14.77% developed osteonecrosis, both events being much greater than for non-BP patients. Some clinical researchers have suggested that the development of osteonecrosis in conjunction with dental implants might be a side effect of treatment with oral or IV bisphosphonates, and the prevalence of BRONJ or MORNJ is persistent during and after the conclusion of therapy. Thus, the implication is that BP therapy may have a potentiating effect on peri-implantitis and implant loss. In contrast, others have found that the prevalence of implant failure was minimal in patients using oral and IV bisphosphonates and that dental implants *can* osseointegrate and be functionally stable, particularly with oral bisphosphonate use [13].

The overall conclusion is that the dentist must exercise caution when planning dental implant surgery in patients undergoing bisphosphonate therapy because of the risk of developing BRONJ (MRONJ) as well as failure of the implant, particularly for patients undergoing IV therapy. The consensus is that dentists treating patients who have taken oral BPs for less than four years and have none of the risk factors indicated above may not need to make alterations in the planned surgery. Nevertheless, if a dental implant surgery is proposed, the dentist should provide the patient with informed consent that indicates possible long-term implant failure and the risk, usually low, of developing osteonecrosis of the jaws.

The indications are that there is a greater risk of implant failure for women taking oral BPs and that with long-term users, the treatment should be discontinued for four to six months prior to implant insertion, and for several months after, to allow for the recovery of bone remodeling [14]. In the case of patients who have taken oral BP for less than four years but have concomitantly taken corticosteroids or antiangiogenic medications, or for patients who have taken oral BP for more than four years with or without any concomitant medical therapy, discontinuation of these drugs should be considered for at least two months and preferably four to six months prior to surgery provided that systemic conditions permit interruption of therapy. BP therapy should not be restarted until osseous healing has occurred. Further, implant patients undergoing bisphosphonate therapy should be followed for long periods because the development of osteonecrosis can be a late complication, and the follow-up period must be extended to detect late-developing signs and symptoms [3–5].

Antibiotics

Interestingly, it has been suggested that patients who developed BRONJ associated with dental implants should undergo a long-term treatment with doxycycline (100–200 mg/d), and the implants should be removed only if the antibiotic therapy fails to alleviate the signs and symptoms of BRONJ/MRONJ.

It was mentioned in Chapter 4 that at least one retrospective cohort study concluded that antibiotics significantly reduced the failure of dental implants under ordinary conditions. Further, it was found that single-dose preoperative antibiotics and preoperative and postoperative antibiotics had similar effects on dental implant failures and infections. Although many dentists are reluctant to prescribe antibiotics unless there are clear indications for their use, antibiotics should be efficacious when there are indications of peri-mucositis or peri-implantitis or if there is a risk of such conditions developing [15].

Implant Failures

Atypical implant failures do occur in situations when there appear to be no contributing factors. An example of this is shown in Fig. 15.3a,b:

(a)   (b)

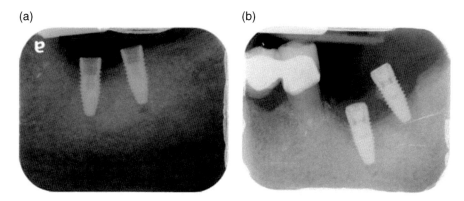

Figure 15.3   (a) Post-operative radiograph. (b) 4 month post-operative radiograph.

In this particular case, an atypical early implant failure occurred which could not be ascribed to any particular cause. There was complete loss of the implant within five days of the situation in Fig. 15.3b. Follow-up radiographs and clinical examination showed no indications of infection at the implant site. Further, there was no indication of epithelial downgrowth surrounding the implant at any time, and no soft-tissue residue was noted on the extruded implant. After adequate healing time for the implant site, the lost implant was replaced by one with a coarser thread and, following successful osseointegration, restoration was completed.

Failures also occur due to causes such as peri-implantitis that develop some time after implant placement and restoration. This is shown in the following example.

An implant was placed for a patient with good quality bone and no obvious intrinsic or extrinsic risk factors, Fig. 15.4a. After placement, the implant was allowed to osseointegrate for a period of six months and then was restored with cement-retained PFM crown. Despite apparently satisfactory oral hygiene practices by the patient, a one year-follow-up after placement indicated that peri-implantitis had developed, (Fig. 15.4b).

Careful clinical examination suggested that several factors might have contributed to the development of peri-implantitis, notably:

- Overloading of the restored implant
- The presence of cement/cement residue within the sulcus
- Inadequate oral hygiene
- Bacterial ingress into the sulcus

The remedial treatment regimen for this situation was:

1. Occlusal adjustment and elimination of bruxism as a contributing factor
2. Deep scaling and irrigation

(a)   (b)

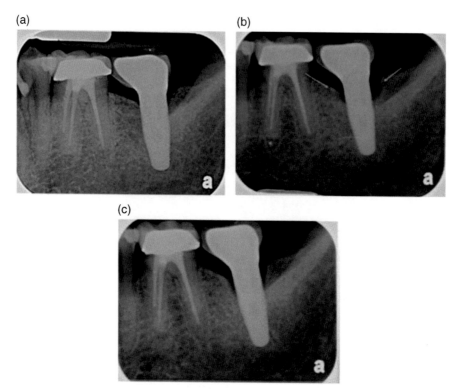

(c)

Figure 15.4 (a) Restoration of the abutment by a cement-retained PFM crown. (b) One-year follow-up radiograph showing peri-implantitis. (c) 5-year post-operative radiograph after remedial treatment.

3. Localized and systemic antibiotic therapy
4. Restoration removal and placement of a healing abutment
5. Careful oral hygiene instruction with follow-up on a regular basis.

In more severe cases, where there is greater loss of bone around the implant, then surgical intervention may be necessary. This approach might involve raising a flap, debriding the implant, decontamination with a laser and, often, a bone graft with membrane coverage.

Saving the Failing Implant

Clearly, in order to avoid implant failure, the dentist should discuss risk factors that can limit the implant success with the patient. Most of these factors have already been addressed in this chapter and the dentist should pay careful attention to any change in the patient's medical condition or medications that can affect healing and osseointegration. Stressing the importance of good oral hygiene is also key to avoiding implant problems. Brushing twice daily and rinsing with an antibacterial mouthwash can help maintain healthy gingivae and avoid bacterial infections during osseointegration [16].

Unfortunately, peri-implantitis and peri-implant bone loss are far more difficult to deal with than total implant loss, if only because the success of the remedial treatment is not particularly predictable. If the progressive loss of osse-ointegration is due to malocclusion, heavy occlusion or severe bruxism, then simple restorative treatments can usually alleviate the issue. In particular, an initial approach should be to remove the restoration and place a cover screw or healing abutment to allow the tissues inflammation to subside.

If there is progressive bone loss due to peri-implantitis, (see Fig. 15.5a,b), then it may be possible to place a bone graft to improve the bone surrounding the implant site. It is important to note that grafting around an existing implant clinically does not observe a high success rate. There are many techniques to clean and decontaminate the implant surface. These techniques include the use of chlorohexidine, phosphoric acid, lasers, titanium brushes, and plasty or polishing and smoothing of the implant surface. If *in situ* grafting is undertaken, it is essential that the patient eliminate any risk factors that may impact the long-term success of the implant.

(a)   (b)

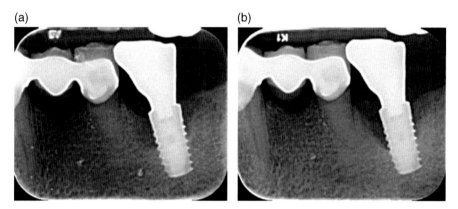

Figure 15.5   (a) Restored implant post-op. (b) Progressive post-op. periodontal problem.

Treating the peri-implantitis and possibly employing a bone graft would be essential to save the implant. This procedure is outlined in the following case.

A typically encountered problem is when a patient presents with chronic gingival irritation on distal of previously placed implant which has resulted in marked bone loss, (Fig. 15.6a). After the restoration was removed to gain access (Fig. 15.6b), a flap was raised, and the implant surface was debrided manually and irrigated with chlorhexidine. Thereafter, a CO_2 laser was used to initially clean the titanium surface followed by treatment with 50% phosphoric acid solution to further clean the surface. There are, of course, several different options for cleansing and decontaminating the implant surface but the approach we routinely adopt has proved to be the most convenient for our purposes.

After preparation of the implant surface, mineralized allograft was placed followed by a resorbable collagen membrane, (Fig. 15.6c). PTFE sutures were used to close the site.

After sufficient healing of the treated site, a new zirconia restoration was placed at five months post-grafting, (Fig. 15.6d).

At the two-year follow-up, it can be seen that the implant was stable with no tissue inflammation and the presence of mature bone was detected radiographically, (Fig. 15.6e).

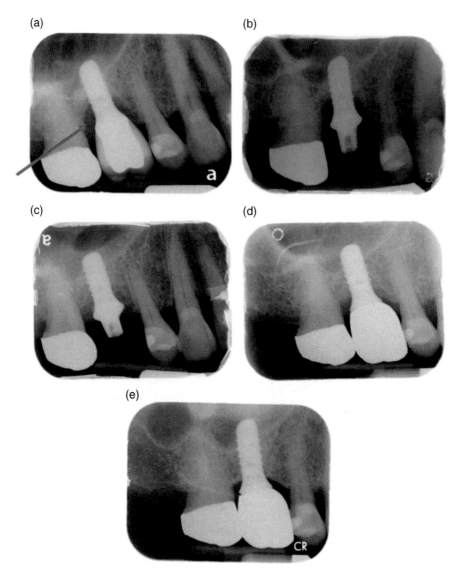

Figure 15.6 (a) Bone loss resulting from chronic gingival irritation. (b) Restoration removed. (c) Mineralized allograft and a resorbable collagen membrane in place. (d) New zirconia crown placed on the implant at 5 months post-grafting. (e) Two-year follow-up radiograph.

Conclusions

Although the implant procedure is quite predictable and has a high success rate, there are risk factors and complications. The main risk factors include the patient's medical history, bone quality, and parafunctional habits. Implant complications can either be biological or mechanical. One of the most common biological complications is fibrous encapsulation. Fibrous encapsulation is when the implant does not integrate to the bone. This can be caused for a variety of reasons but often the reason cannot be pinpointed. Peri-implant mucositis is inflammation of the tissues around the implant. Peri-implantitis is bone loss around the implant. Mechanical complications include screw loosening, screw fracture, and implant fracture.

References

1. Moy, P.K., Medina, D., Shetty, V. et al. (2005). Dental implant failure rates and associated risk factors. *Int. J. Oral Maxillofac. Implants* 20 (4): 569–577.
2. Chrcanovic, B.R., Kisch, J., and Albrektsson, T. (2016). Factors influencing early dental implant failures. *J. Dent. Res.* 95 (9): 995–1002.
3. Paquette, D.W., Brodala, N., and Williams, R.C. (2006). Risk factors for endosseous dental implant failure. *Dent. Clin. North Am.* 50 (3): 361–374.
4. Sverzut, A.T., Stabile, G.A.V., Moraes, M. et al. (2008). The influence of tobacco on early dental implant failure. *J. Oral Maxillofac. Surg.* 66 (5): 1004–1009.
5. Levin, L., Ofec, R., Grossmann, Y., and Anner, R. (2011). Periodontal disease as a risk for dental implant failure over time: a long-term historical cohort study. *J. Clin. Periodontol.* 38: 732–737.
6. Jemt, T., Olsson, M., Renouard, F. et al. (2016). Early implant failures related to individual surgeons: an analysis covering 11,074 operations performed during 28 years. *Clin. Implant Dent. Relat. Res.* 18 (5): 861–872.
7. Pratt, L.A., Brody, D.J. and Gu, Q. (2011). Antidepressant Use in Persons Aged 12 and Over: United States, 2005–2008. *NCHS Data Brief* (76): 1–8.
8. Tolemeo, P.G., Lee, J.S., and Miller, E.J. Jr. (2016). Selective serotonin inhibitors and dental implants osseointegration. *Journal of Oral and Maxillofacial Surgery* 74 (9): 55–56.
9. Hakam, A.E., Duarte, P.M., Vila, M.P. et al. (2020). Effects of different antidepressant classes on dental implant failure: a retrospective clinical study. *J. Periodontol.* https://doi.org/10.1002/JPER.19-0714. Online ahead of print.
10. Diab, D.L. and Watts, N.B. (2012). Bisphosphonates in the treatment of osteoporosis. *Endocrinol. and Metab. Clin. North Am.* 41 (3): 487–506.
11. Ruggiero, S.L., Dodson, T.B., Fantasia, J. et al. (2014). American Association of Oral and Maxillofacial Surgeons position paper on medication-related osteonecrosis of the jaw – 2014 update. *J. Oral Maxillofac. Surg.* 72 (10): 1938–1956.
12. de-Freitas, N.-R., Lima, L.-B., de-Moura, M.-B. et al. (2016). Bisphosphonate treatment and dental implants: a systematic review. *Med. Oral Pathol. Oral Cir. Bucal.* 21 (5): e644–e651.
13. Chadha, G.K., Ahmadieh, A., Satish Kumar, S. et al. (2013). Osseointegration of dental implants and osteonecrosis of the jaw in patients treated with bisphosphonate therapy: a systematic review. *J. Oral Implantol.* 39 (4): 510–520.
14. Ruggiero, S.L., Dodson, T.B., Fantasia, J. et al. (2014). American Association of Oral and Maxillofacial Surgeons position paper on medication-related osteonecrosis of the jaw-2014 update. *J. Oral Maxillofac. Surg.* 72: 1938–1956.
15. Surapaneni, H., Yalamanchili, P.S., Basha, M.D. et al. (2016). Antibiotics in dental implants: a review of literature. *J. Pharm. Bioallied Sci.* 8 (Suppl 1): S28–S31.
16. Pedrazzi, V., Escobar, E.C., Jr, C. et al. (2014). Antimicrobial mouthrinse use as an adjunct method in peri-implant biofilm control. *Braz. Oral Res.* 28 (Spec Iss 1): 1–9.

16

Economics of Dental Implants

Implant dentistry is well within the scope and capabilities of the general dental practitioner. Not only can implant dentistry be profitable but this well-established approach to dental care is often a superior treatment option where a prosthesis is needed by a patient. According to the American College of Prosthodontics, more than 35 million Americans do not have any teeth, 178 million people in the U.S. are missing at least one tooth [1] and significant numbers of Americans would benefit from dental implant treatment [2, 3]. It was estimated back in 2001 that 300000 to 428000 endosseous dental implants were placed annually in the U.S., and this statistic was projected to grow at ≈12% annually [4]. In fact, the American Dental Association (ADA) [5] has stated that five million dental implants are placed each year by dentists in the U.S.

Establishing and building an implant practice does require thought and planning. However, three things can contribute to future success:

- Marketing
- Staff training
- Gaining experience and expertise through continuing education

It is recommended and important to establish a set of procedures that you will offer to patients. After the proper training, the practice should begin to diagnose and create treatment plans for these procedures.

The first phase of implementing dental implant treatment into the general practice starts with diagnosis. As you train your staff and treatment plans are presented, you will start to achieve some case acceptance.

The ADA Practical Guide to Dental Implants, First Edition. Luigi O. Massa and J. Anthony von Fraunhofer.
© 2021 The American Dental Association. Published 2021 by John Wiley & Sons, Inc.

The second phase of implementing dental implant treatment into general practice is execution while gaining expertise and confidence. Your case acceptance will increase with your growing expertise, experience, and confidence.

The third and final phase of implementing dental implant treatment into general practice is when patients come to your office seeking implant therapy. Many times, you may already have placed and restored an implant on these patients, and they have returned for additional implants to be placed. This cycle may take two to three years to accomplish.

Implant dentistry is the standard of care in many situations and the general dentist should not hesitate to provide this much-needed service if they are comfortable and confident in doing so.

The Dental Implant Practice

Every dental practice is different and there is no "one-size-fits-all" when it comes to running that practice or establishing one that performs dental implants. It goes without saying, practices vary in terms of the number of dentists, staffing, patients, and myriad other factors that contribute to its success, financial and otherwise.

The comments made here are based on a successful multi-location group of one of the author's practices in Texas. Office rent, utilities, staffing costs and other overheads will vary with the location and, likewise, laboratory costs and other overhead items will be dependent on the practice, its facilities and location. The cost breakdowns discussed here are specific to this group of practices.

Many of the costs cited below may be specific to laboratory and other fees current in Texas. Further, the group practice also owns CT scanners, together with a large central laboratory, where many items such as osteotomy guides and other facets of treatment are fabricated. These facets of the practice do have a major bearing on the costs of the implant dentistry treatment provided within the author's practices.

The costs of implant kits and associated armamentarium given here are those for 2020 and may change over next few years, depending on the overall economy and that pertaining to dentistry as a profession.

Basic Considerations

A general practitioner has a set of procedures that are performed daily. One of these procedures is the single-tooth crown. It has already been stated (Chapter 6) that in restorative dentistry, the crown generally meets the following criteria:

- Long-term success rate
- Predictable outcome
- Low-stress procedure
- Profitability

These same criteria are met and often exceeded with implant dentistry.

Consider the basic fees associated with a single tooth crown.

1. Supply costs ($50–$75)
    a. Burs
    b. Custom or stock tray
    c. Impression material
2. Laboratory costs ($100–$200)

Assuming a usual and customary patient crown fee of $1000, the basic fees account for 15–27% of the patient fee.

The guiding principle for our implant practice is to base the single implant treatment on the cost of a standard three-unit bridge. Philosophically, we would like our patients to choose the best option based on outcomes and not on fees. The standard usual and customary fee for a three-unit bridge in our practice is roughly $3250 and so our fee for an implant is $3250. This "implant package" includes both tooth extraction if necessary, together with bone grafting at the time of implant placement if necessary. This charge also includes the final abutment and final restoration (generally a screw-retained restoration). However, it does not include any pre-implant ridge augmentation or an interim restoration if deemed necessary. Pre-implant ridge augmentation would consist of guided-bone regeneration to increase the width or height of the ridge prior to implant placement. It would also consist of socket preservation grafting if using a staged approach to implant placement.

Cost Breakdowns

The authors would like to stress that the cost breakdowns are those for the region in which they practice, namely South Texas, and for the instrumentation they routinely use. Costs will vary across the U.S. depending upon numerous economic factors as well as with the instrumentation selected by the individual practitioner. Consequently, the cost breakdowns indicated here should be considered as guides rather than definitive statements regarding costs and treatment charges.

The Single Implant

In most single implant cases, the same basic fees apply:

1. Implant costs
    a. Single implant kit: $225–$450[1]
    b. Graft material (average per site): $30–$50
2. Supplies ($30–$50)
    a. Custom or stock tray
    b. Impression material
3. Laboratory charges ($250–$450)
    a. Soft-tissue model
    b. Lab analog
    c. Abutment/titanium base
    d. Zirconia restoration

Total cost of supplies/laboratory fees: $535–$1000. These laboratory fees should be comparable for all implant procedures.

Assuming a usual and customary implant patient fee of $3250, the basic fees account for 16%–30% of the patient fee. This meets the percentages associated with a single tooth crown.

The Mandibular Overdenture (Two to Three Implants)

- Two to three implants: $225–450 each
- Two to three abutments/attachments: $150
- Cast metal frame: $150
- Denture: $350

Total average cost: ~$1250–$2300

Assuming a usual and customary mandibular overdenture patient fee of ~$8000, the basic fees account for 16%–29% of the patient fee.

The Maxillary Overdenture (Four Implants)

- Four implants: $225–$450 ea.
- Four abutments/attachments: $150
- Cast metal frame: $150
- Denture: $350

Total average cost: ~$2000–$2900

In our practices, assuming a usual and customary patient maxillary overdenture fee of $12 000, the basic fees account for 17–24% of the patient fee.

Comparable cost analyses can be made for every dental implant procedure. The bottom line is that implant dentistry can, and should be, profitable for the dentist while also providing the best possible treatment for the patient.

The capital cost of advanced technology such as CT radiography and other equipment undoubtedly is high but is essential for an effective and efficient dental implant practice. Such equipment is unlikely to be available or within the operating budget of a fledgling implant practice. Accordingly, it should be possible and sensible to arrange for different practices to share the cost of equipment. Shared major equipment items is an approach adopted by many practices and is both cost-effective and a major factor in operational efficiency.

Financing

With today's technology, many prostheses such as complete dentures are less desirable, and implant-retained bridges can replace removable (and fixed) partial dentures. A well-organized, modern, and innovative practice can make these services available and affordable.

Unfortunately, some dental insurance plans will not cover the costs of implants, regardless of the patient's needs. This can create financial problems for the patient desiring optimal care while preventing the dentist from providing the best treatment for a variety of clinical issues.

Insurance concerns result in many patients being unable to afford or be reluctant to undertake implant dentistry. In many cases, patients cannot or will not pay what might appear to be a much higher fee for an implant-retained prosthesis compared to the cost of conventional treatment, however unsatisfactory the latter might be. This is where financing partners can be helpful to both patient and the dental provider.

Many financial institutions currently or potentially can finance the cost of implant dentistry throughout the U.S. The dentist about to embark on an implant practice should establish contact with suitable financial institutions so that prospective patients are able to know the immediate and deferred costs before treatment is started.

Conclusions

Analyzing the costs involved with performing implant procedures is an important exercise. If a practitioner decides to provide these services, it is beneficial to compare the costs involved to that of a commonly performed procedure like a full coverage crown. Implant dentistry meets many of the same criteria as the crown procedure such as long-term success rate, predictable outcome, low-stress procedure for the dentist and profitability.

Note

1. Depending upon the manufacturer, the cover screw, healing abutment, transfer and final abutment may be included in several available implant kits and, therefore, there may be no charge for these items when used by the clinician and laboratory.

References

1. American College of Prosthodontists (2020). Facts and figures. https://www.gotoapro.org/facts-figures/ (accessed 31 July 2020).
2. Meskin, L.H. and Brown, L.J. (1988). Prevalence and patterns of tooth loss in U.S. employed adult and senior populations, 1985-86. *J. Dent. Educ.* 52: 686–691.
3. Harvey, C. and Kelly, J.E. (1981). Decayed, missing and filled teeth among persons 1-74 years, United States. *Vital Health Stat.* 11 (223): 1–55.
4. Millennium Research Group (2001). U.S. markets for dental implants 2001: executive summary. *Implant Dent.* 10: 234–237.
5. American Dental Association Patient Education Center (2014). *Dental Implants.* Chicago, IL: ADA.

17

Maintaining Dental Implants

In the early decades of the twentieth century, it was commonplace for people to have all their teeth extracted and replaced by dentures on the principle that "If you have all your teeth extracted, you will no longer have any problems with them." Whereas the extracted teeth are now surgical scrap and can no longer present problems for the patient, the dental profession is aware that edentulism presents a host of oral and systemic problems and does not cure or prevent oral disease. In fact, the opposite is usually the case.

Unfortunately, whereas replacing missing or failing dentition with implants may provide an immediate solution to complete or partial edentulism, many patients do not appreciate that continuing care is mandatory for the health and longevity of implants. In fact, it is a reasonable assertion that if the implant patient had paid as much attention to oral hygiene, they might still be dentate.

There is no question that oral hygiene procedures with dental implants can be tedious, but it is critical to long-term oral health and survival of the implant, and both the patient and the dental professional must exercise considerable effort to ensure the success and longevity of the implant.

Preventing Implant Failures

Implant dentistry has possibly become the most important treatment regimen in restorative dentistry because of the extremely high success rates of long-term dental implant survival and their restorations. Consequently, increasing numbers of patients select dental implants as a treatment option.

However, the dental team can be presented with challenges in situations when patients are reluctant to undertake even basic oral hygiene procedures. Part of

The ADA Practical Guide to Dental Implants, First Edition. Luigi O. Massa and J. Anthony von Fraunhofer.
© 2021 The American Dental Association. Published 2021 by John Wiley & Sons, Inc.

Table 17.1 Factors in the success or failure of implants.

Surgical site
Surgical technique
Type of surgery (one- or two-stage)
Immediate or delayed implant placement
Bone augmentation
Insertion torque
Implant length and width
Implant surface texture and coatings
Collar design
Implant-abutment connection design
Systemic health factors
Infection
Occlusal stresses
Oral hygiene

the challenge is that the focus of implant dentistry has changed from simply achieving osseointegration, which is now highly predictable, to the long-term maintenance of the health of the peri-implant hard and soft tissues. This requires appropriate professional care, patient cooperation, and effective home care. Thus, in order to ensure a successful outcome for an implant and its restoration, patients must accept the responsibility of being co-therapists in maintenance therapy and, consequently, the dental team must screen potential implant patients to ensure that these are achievable goals. Typically, diagnosis and treatment planning based on a risk–benefit analysis should be performed after a thorough medical, dental, head-and-neck, psychological and radiographic examination as well as a temporomandibular joint health evaluation.

Failure of implants was discussed in Chapter 15 and it was indicated that the predominant causes of failures are infection, peri-implantitis, inadequate or failure of initial osseointegration and, ultimately, loss of osseointegration, see Table 17.1. Two of these causes are related to oral hygiene while the last is predominantly caused by masticatory stresses and bruxism. The effect of unbalanced malocclusion on implants is discussed later in this chapter.

Many of the factors possibly contributing to implant failure have been discussed in previous chapters.

Indicators of Implant Problems

There is a steadily growing literature on the monitoring of the stability and osseointegration of dental implants and, increasingly, electronic and other non-invasive technologies are being recommended for this important task [1–6]. However, possibly the best indicator for the diagnosis and/or prediction of implant failure is the presence of mobility. In contrast to a natural tooth with a periodontal ligament, osseointegrated implants should exhibit no clinically detectable movement and, therefore, healthy implants should appear to be nonmobile. There should be **no mobility** even in the presence of peri-implant bone loss provided there is still an adequate amount of supporting integrated alveolar bone.

When monitoring the health of the peri-implant soft tissues, the practitioner and hygienist should be cognizant of changes in soft tissue such as those to color, contour and consistency. The presence of a fistulous tract, for example, could indicate the presence of a pathologic process or impending implant fracture.

The significance of bleeding upon probing around dental implants is still being debated in the literature although it is generally accepted that bleeding upon probing or palpation may be an indication of peri-implant disease [7–9]. This is because bleeding can occur before there are any histological signs of inflammation or it may occur concurrently with other signs of implant failure such as bone loss. However, as discussed below, routine (and, especially, aggressive) probing is not recommended for implant sites.

Radiographic interpretation is probably the most useful clinical parameter for evaluating the status of an endosseous dental implant. Invasion of the biological width and predictable remodeling, e.g., "saucerization," leads to an average marginal bone loss of about 1.5 mm during the first year following prosthetic rehabilitation. This is potentially followed by an average vertical bone loss of 0.2 mm every subsequent year. Thus, if the progressive bone loss around a dental implant exceeds these averages, then this may be taken to be an indicator of an ailing or failing implant. Lastly, during radiographic evaluation, there should be no evidence of peri-implant radiolucency because such a rarefaction usually indicates an active (or past) infection and/or failure of osseointegration or a recurrent cyst.

Natural Teeth vs Implants

Problems can arise with implants because of differences in the periodontal relationship between the gingiva and the structure it attaches to regardless of whether it is a natural tooth or an implant. The most crestal connection of the gingival cuff around both natural teeth and dental implants is the junctional epithelium which functions as a physical barrier to ingress of bacteria (and food debris), thereby limiting or preventing inflammation. However, the junctional epithelium differs between natural teeth and implants with respect to both the orientation of the fibers and the strength of the attachment.

With a natural tooth, the fiber orientation of the gingival cuff is such that it attaches perpendicularly to the long axis of the tooth and functions as a barrier when inserting a periodontal probe within the sulcus. Consequently, the probe tip can be advanced apically until the tip contacts the perpendicular fibers and is halted. This orientation is not seen around implants. In contrast, the gingival fiber orientation is parallel to the implant's long axis. Consequently, when a periodontal probe is inserted into the sulcus, the advancing probe tip can pass between the fibers of the gingival cuff until the crestal bone is reached, and there is no further advancement. The net result is that the peri-implant mucosal seal surrounding an implant may provide a less effective barrier to bacterial plaque than the periodontium surrounding a natural tooth, (Fig. 17.1).

The probing depth around dental implants is related to the thickness and type of mucosa surrounding the implant and, usually, the healthy peri-implant sulcus ranges from 1.3 to 3.8 mm, i.e., greater than the ideal sulcus depths for natural

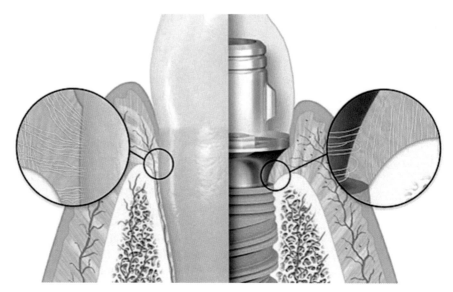

Figure 17.1   Periodontal attachment to the implant body (*Source*: Courtesy of Nobel Biocare).

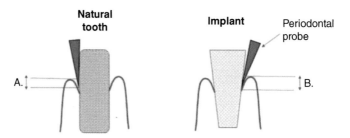

Probe/pocket depth for implant B > than depth A for a natural tooth

Figure 17.2   Relative probe depths for teeth and implants.

teeth. It should also be noted that probing to determine pocket depths, the traditional means of evaluating "periodontal health" can be misleading with implants. This is because of the geometric differences between a natural tooth and an implant. The former has a quasi-parallel-sided crown-to-apex profile whereas implants are pyramidal and, due to these geometric differences, probe depths for the latter can be misleading, (see Fig. 17.2).

It follows from this that during post-operative and routine hygiene appointments, peri-implant periodontal probing should be performed only where there are signs of infection. Such indications include swelling, bleeding on palpation or probing, exudate, inflamed peri-implant soft tissue and/or radiographic evidence of peri-implant alveolar bone loss. The "take-home" message is that routine periodontal probing of dental implants is inadvisable because it could damage the inherently weak epithelial attachment around the implant and possibly create a pathway for the ingress of periodontal pathogens. Thus, in the authors' opinion, the best indicator for evaluating an unhealthy site might be probing data gathered longitudinally.

It is also important to note that plastic probes should be used when investigating the crevicular depth around dental implants. This will avoid galvanic interaction between stainless steel probes and the titanium of the implant body, i.e., prevent electric "shocks" for the patient.

Another factor is that the gingival tissue surrounding dental implants is less vascularized than with natural teeth which, combined with the parallel-oriented collagen fibers adjacent to the implant body, renders the dental implant more vulnerable to bacterial insult. Consequently, any disruption of the gingival fibers attached to the implant, for example, by aggressive probing or mechanical cleansing devices can increase the susceptibility to the ingress of bacteria.

Hygiene Instrumentation

The literature clearly indicates that bacterial plaque not only leads to gingivitis and periodontitis but also can induce the development of peri-implantitis. Thus, personal oral hygiene must begin at the time of dental implant placement and should be modified as required using various adjunctive aids for oral hygiene to effectively clean the altered morphology of the peri-implant region before, during and after implant placement and its restoration.

The clinical use of metallic instruments, typically stainless steel, should be limited to natural teeth and not used to probe or scale dental implants. The rationale for this well-documented [10–12], and a frequently expressed warning is because the stainless steel used to manufacture dental and surgical instruments is so hard it can scratch, abrade or contaminate the implant surface. Further, stainless steel instruments may strip off any surface treatment of the implant body such as a hydroxyapatite (HA) coating [13] or cause a galvanic reaction at the implant-abutment interface if the implant body is exposed. The possibility of galvanic interactions is an important consideration since it has been shown that galvanic corrosion between different metals (titanium and stainless steel) delayed healing in a mandibular fracture [14] and that between a precious metal crown and a titanium implant caused failure of that implant [15].

In fact, a variety of materials have been used for fabricating manual periodontal scalers intended for cleaning dental implants, including various resins, Teflon polytetrafluoroethylene (PTFE), gold-plated metals and even wood. However, when using gold-plated curettes, manufacturers advise against sharpening these instruments because the gold surface coating can be chipped or damaged to expose the hard surface of the base metal substrate of the scaling instrument.

Other cleaning armamentarium contra-indicated for use with dental implants are air-powder abrasion units, flour of pumice polish or sonic and ultrasonic scaling units. The scaler tips of ultrasonic, piezo or sonic units may damage the implant surface, causing micro-roughness and facilitating plaque accumulation. It is also possible for the scaler tips to cause gouging or deep scratching of the implant's polished collar. Some clinicians advocate placing a plastic sleeve over the tip when using ultrasonic scaling on dental implants since this approach apparently provides effective cleaning while reducing the risk of damage to the implant.

Air-powder polishing units should be avoided during hygiene appointments involving implants, again to reduce the risk of damage to the implant surface as well as damage and possibly complete stripping of any surface coating. This stripping can still occur even if the relatively benign, abrasion-free baking soda powder is used in these units. Additionally, the air pressure used in such units can sometimes be so great that it may detach the soft-tissue connection with the coronal portion of the implant, leading to emphysema [16].

It is safe, however, to polish the surfaces of titanium and titanium alloy implant surfaces using a rubber cup and a non-abrasive polishing paste or even a gauze strip and tin oxide.

Patient-Applied Oral Hygiene Measures

Notwithstanding the importance of regular professional dental hygiene care of implants, the home-care techniques for maintaining the health of endosseous dental implants are also crucial to long-term implant success. Accordingly, as with dentate patients, the implant patient's home-care requirements should be individually tailored according to his or her individual needs. The latter are based on the location and angulation of the dental implants, the position and length of transmucosal abutments, the type of prosthesis, and the manual dexterity of the patient. Patients should be taught the modified Bass technique of brushing using a soft-bristled toothbrush with a medium-sized head [17–19].

As with natural dentition, adjunctive cleaning aids such as flossing are still valuable. The use of interdental brushes by implant patients should be encouraged only after they have received instruction on their proper use. In the authors' opinion, the plastic-coated wire brush is the only type that should be used to clean around and adjacent to dental implant in order to avoid scratching the implant surface. The routine (and regular) use of interproximal brushes should be encouraged since they can penetrate up to 3 mm into a gingival sulcus or pocket and may effectively clean the peri-implant sulcus. A recent review [20] has clearly shown that interdental cleaning is correlated with increased periodontal health and patients with severe periodontal disease could show additional oral health benefits by increasing the frequency of interdental cleaning. In addition to mechanical plaque control, daily rinses using 0.1% chlorhexidine gluconate or anti-bacterial mouth washes are useful oral hygiene adjuncts for preventive maintenance.

Recently, there has been increased attention paid in media advertising regarding the use of automated mechanical toothbrushes for teeth cleansing and improved oral hygiene. These devices may have rotary, reciprocating or sonic action. However, despite the advertising onslaught, the key to the effectiveness of mechanical toothbrushes is proper instruction on their use and then diligent daily use by the implant patient.

The other popular types of cleansing device are the oral irrigators, also known as water picks and water jets, which can be used with or without the addition of antimicrobial solutions. Careful use of these devices will dilute and sluice away plaque-generated acids, food debris and bacteria, particularly accumulations from interproximal areas and in some subgingival pockets. On the other hand, patients should not only be instructed on their proper use but also be warned that some oral irrigators can be "wound up" to deliver water jets under high pressure. Operating oral irrigators at very high pressures can not only drive debris and bacteria into the sulcus but also damage the epithelial attachment to the implant.

It follows from this discussion that the long-term success of dental implants requires patient–clinician cooperation, education and collaboration as well as continuing attention to oral hygiene on a daily basis using the appropriate armamentarium.

Conclusions

Continuing care is mandatory for the long-term success of dental implants. Routine dental visits allow the practitioner to monitor the implant and the prosthesis. The most common methods to monitor the implant are radiographic evaluation and clinical evaluation. Tracking bone levels radiographically over time is a key indicator to the stability of the implant. Likewise, clinical evaluation of the hard and soft tissues is a key indicator. The practitioner should evaluate for inflammation, bleeding upon palpation and presence of purulence. In addition, the patient's home care is one of the most important factors to ensure the success of a dental implant. The patient should be instructed on the appropriate home-care routine which should consist of a combination of the following: brushing, interproximal cleaning, and irrigation.

References

1. Dariob, L.J., Cucchiarob, P.J., and Deluziob, A.J. (2002). Electronic monitoring of dental implant osseointegration. *J. Am. Dent. Assoc.* 133 (4): 483–490.
2. Salvi, G.E. and Lang, N.P. (2004). Diagnostic parameters for monitoring peri-implant conditions. *Int. J. Oral Maxillofac. Implants* 19 (7): 116–127.
3. Rizzo, P. (2020). A review on the latest advancements in the non-invasive evaluation/monitoring of dental and trans-femoral implants. *Biomed. Eng. Lett.* 10: 83–102.
4. Sjöström, M., Lundgren, S., Nilson, H. et al. (2005). Monitoring of implant stability in grafted bone using resonance frequency analysis: a clinical study from implant placement to 6 months of loading. *Int. J. Oral Maxillofac. Surg.* 34 (1): 45–51.
5. Tarawali, K. (2015). Maintenance and monitoring of dental implants in general dental practice. *Dent. Update* 42 (6): 513–514. 517–518.
6. Ward, S.T., Czuszak, C.A., Thompson, A.L. et al. (2012). Assessment and maintenance of dental implants: clinical and knowledge-seeking practices of dental hygienists. *J. Dent. Hyg.* 86 (2): 104–110.
7. Farina, R., Filippi, M., Brazzioli, J. et al. (2016). Bleeding on probing around dental implants: a retrospective study of associated factors. *J. Clin. Periodontol.* 44: 115–122.
8. Magnuson, B., Harsono, M., Stark, P.C. et al. (2013). Comparison of the effect of two interdental cleaning devices around implants on the reduction of bleeding: a 30-day randomized clinical trial. *Compend. Contin. Educ. Dent.* 34 (8): 2–7.
9. Gerber, J.A., Tan, W.C., Balmer, T.E. et al. (2009). Bleeding on probing and pocket probing depth in relation to probing pressure and mucosal health around oral implants. *Clin. Oral Implants Res.* 20 (1): 75–78.
10. Dmytiyk, J.J., Fox, S.C., and Moriarty, J.D. (1990). The effects of scaling titanium implant surfaces with metal and plastic instruments on cell attachment. *J. Periodontol.* 61 (8): 491–496.

11. de Almeida Curylofo, F., Barbosa, A., Roselino, A.L. et al. (2012). Instrumentation of dental implants: a literature review. *RSBO* 10 (1): 82–88.

12. Louropoulou, A., Slot, D.E., and Van der Weijden, F. (2015). Influence of mechanical instruments on the biocompatibility of titanium dental implants surfaces: a systematic review. *Clin. Oral Implants Res.* 26 (7): 841–850.

13. Nasar, A. (2019). Hydroxyapatite and its coatings in dental implants. In: *Applications of Nanocomposite Materials in Dentistry*, Woodhead Publishing Series in Biomaterials (eds. A.M. Asiri, Inamuddin and A. Mohammed), 145–160. Cambridge, UK: Woodhead Publishing.

14. Steiner, M., von Fraunhofer, J.A., and Mascaro, J. (1981). The role of corrosion in inhibiting the healing of a mandibular fracture. *J. Oral Surg.* 39: 140–143.

15. von Fraunhofer, J.A., Kohut, D., and Mackie, K.D. (2017). Implant failure caused by galvanic corrosion. *EC Dent. Sci.* 12 (5): 196–203.

16. S-Tak, L., Subu, M.G., and Kwon, T.-G. (2018). Emphysema following air-powder abrasive treatment for peri-implantitis. *Maxillofac. Plast. Reconstr. Surg.* 40: 12–17.

17. Kracher, C.M., Smith, W.S., and Schmeling, W. (2010). Oral health maintenance of dental implants. *Dent. Assist.* 79 (2): 27–35.

18. Swierkot, K., Brusius, M., Leismann, D. et al. (2013). Manual versus sonic-powered toothbrushing for plaque reduction in patients with dental implants: an explanatory randomised controlled trial. *Eur. J. Oral Implantol.* 6 (2): 133–144.

19. Clark, D. and Levin, L. (2016). Dental implant management and maintenance: how to improve long-term implant success. *Quintessence Int.* 47 (5): 417–423.

20. Marchesan, J.T., Morelli, T., Moss, K. et al. (2019). Interdental cleaning is associated with decreased oral disease prevalence. *J. Dent. Res.* 97: 773–7788.

Restoring Dental Implants

After placement of the dental implant and successful osseointegration, undertaking restoration of the implant is a multi-step process.

Step 1

Place and tighten the fixture mount/transfer to use as the transfer, Fig. A.1a, b, with the flat side of the post, oriented towards the buccal:

The fixture mount/transfer should be prepared by covering the screw access hole with wax:

(a) (b)

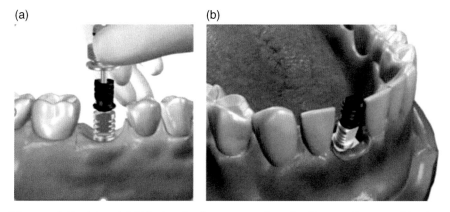

Figures A.1 (a) and (b) Placing the fixture mount/transfer (*Source*: Courtesy of Implant Direct).

The ADA Practical Guide to Dental Implants, First Edition. Luigi O. Massa and J. Anthony von Fraunhofer.
© 2021 The American Dental Association. Published 2021 by John Wiley & Sons, Inc.

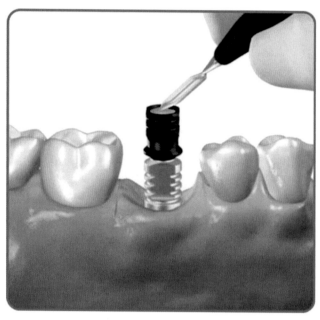

Figure A.2 Covering the screw access hole with wax (*Source*: Courtesy of Implant Direct).

Step 2

Inject impression material around the fixture/transfer mount and press the tray down firmly and allow to set before removing it:

(a)   (b)

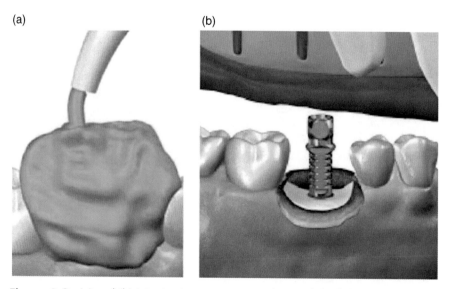

Figure A.3 (a) and (b) Injecting impression material around the fixture/transfer mount and removing the impression tray (*Source*: Courtesy of Implant Direct).

Note that the dentist should closely monitor the level of implant impressioning. This has several advantages:

1. Allows for more versatility in restoration.
2. Allows for custom abutment fabrication, screw-retained crown fabrication, or stock abutment use.
3. Margins should be 0.5–1 mm sub-gingival in the final restoration.
4. Facilitates accurate cement clean-up – this is an important consideration since cement residue is a major contributing factor in peri-implantitis.

Step 2a

If digital impressioning is to be performed, the following sequence should be adopted:

a. Remove the healing abutment.
b. Scan the tissue profile.
c. Place the scan adapter.
d. Scan.

Step 3

Replace the healing collar or two-piece cover screw and extender using a hex driver.

(a)

(b)

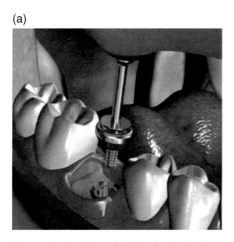 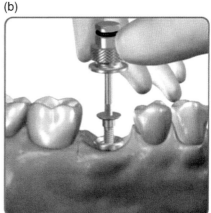

Figure A.4   (a) and (b) Replacing healing collar (*Source*: Courtesy of Implant Direct).

Step 4

Send the impression, fixture/transfer mount, bite, and opposing arch to the dental lab.

Appendix B

Abutments

The design and characteristics of abutments were discussed in Chapter 3, but their clinical use was touched upon only briefly. They are discussed in more detail here.

The role of the implant abutment, in simple terms, is to provide a screwed or threaded connection between the implant and the crown of the prosthetic tooth. Other than the various materials used to produce the abutment, there are two additional categories: stock (prefabricated) dental abutments and custom abutments.

However, central to the selection of an abutment, as discussed elsewhere, is the emergence profile. This is usually defined as the contour of a tooth or restoration where it emerges from the bone in relation to the gingiva, but it can also describe the contour of an abutment where it ascends from the implant platform. Together with the size/diameter of the implant, a determinant of the emergence profile is the type of abutment and the restoration. The objective during restoration of implants is to achieve a natural emergence profile to avoid the restoration trapping plaque, causing difficulties in maintaining good oral hygiene and to avoid an unnatural appearance to the restoration.

Healing Abutments

Healing abutments are designed to create and optimize an emergence profile.

These designs will facilitate optimal soft-tissue contouring during healing following implant placement. They are commonly replaced by permanent abutments during the implant restoration process.

The ADA Practical Guide to Dental Implants, First Edition. Luigi O. Massa and J. Anthony von Fraunhofer.
© 2021 The American Dental Association. Published 2021 by John Wiley & Sons, Inc.

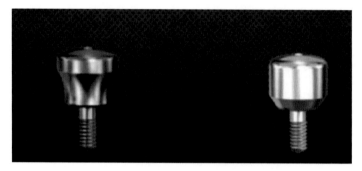

Figure B.1   Stock healing abutments (*Source:* Courtesy of Implant Direct).

Categories of Abutments

There are, broadly, four categories of abutments:

1. Temporary abutments
2. Stock (prefabricated) abutments
   i.   Straight
   ii. Angled
   iii. Straight/Angled zirconia
   iv. Engaging/Non-engaging
3. UCLA gold cast-to abutments
4. Custom abutments
   i.   Ti-Base
   ii. Zr-base.

Temporary Abutments

Temporary abutments are available in two broad styles, namely plastic or titanium, and are either engaging or non-engaging. Their primary use is to retain and support screw-retained temporary restorations prior to final restoration of the implant.

Stock Abutments

Stock or prefabricated abutments are available in a variety of collar heights based on the tissue height, but the other selection criteria include being straight or angled, having a titanium (Ti) or zirconia (Zr) base as well as engaging or non-engaging. The overall purpose of the stock abutment is to provide an easy and user-friendly device that saves time and is more economical than custom-made implant abutments. They are usually used for cement-retained restorations.

Stock abutments are available either as straight or manufactured at a certain angle depending on the location of the dental implant and the requirements of each specific patient. Stock abutments are usually more acceptable for locations that are less visible because the gingival tissue will comply to the shape of the abutment during and after healing following implant placement. This facet of their use may be a limitation within the anterior region.

Engaging abutments have a deep internal connection which makes them suitable for single-unit applications and all cement-retained multi-unit cases. Non-engaging abutments have a shallow internal connection which permits some divergence of the implants with screw-retained multi-unit cases.

Generally, stock abutments are torqued to 35 Ncm during seating and, commonly, crowns are cemented in place onto the abutments. However, stock abutments can be converted to accommodate screw-retained restorations by creating a screw hole and then indirectly cementing the restoration. It is also possible to adjust and/or customize stock abutments.

The primary advantage of stock abutments is their lower cost compared to other abutments but there are certain disadvantages to their use. In particular, because they are a "one size fits all" option when it comes to the emergence profile. Consequently, margins may have an unnatural appearance and often they may be too sub-gingival on the mesial and distal aspects and this can lead to a sub-gingival cement junction. Further, when a stock abutment is used in a more visible location in the mouth, i.e. more anteriorly, it can be difficult to create a natural-appearing emergence of the crown contour relative to the adjacent teeth. An additional issue with a stock abutment is that the final placement of the crown may not be as precise or as easily controlled as the dentist might wish because final placement is dependent on the height and depth of the abutment *and* the implant.

UCLA Abutments

The UCLA Abutment is a castable abutment available with a machined base and is fabricated from metals/alloys such as titanium (Ti), chromium-cobalt (CrCo), or gold (Au). This abutment has the advantage that it can be used for single- or multi-unit screw- or cement-retained restorations. The UCLA abutment was designed to resolve implant angulation problems and, in some cases, depth problems such as too much or too little with respect to the positioning and placement of the implant.

UCLA abutments are manufactured with a gold internal connection and a wax sleeve to which the lab can wax to and cast a restoration from a high noble alloy or a semi-precious alloy. They are available with engaging or non-engaging internal connections. These abutments are primarily used for screw-retained crowns and bridgework.

Although the castable UCLA abutment can correct angles up to 30° when cast as a custom abutment, under normal circumstances, it is unable to address implant positioning problems as well as those possible with a machined (custom) abutment. Accordingly, the "overcasted" UCLA abutment was developed which has a metal base (Ti, CrCo or Au) with a plastic sleeve that can be overcast to achieve the flexibility of providing a versatile abutment that can satisfy almost every demand possible with a precision close to that of a machined abutment. The term "overcastable" might be more suitable for, and descriptive of, these abutments.

The advantages of the overcasted UCLA abutment include:

a. Corrosion resistance
   i.   Minimized risk of irritation and allergic reactions
   ii. Excellent biocompatibility

    b. Reduced complications with surrounding tissues

    c. Combines a high precision machined interface between the implant and the abutment with the convenience of a castable plastic sleeve

    d. Superior performance compared to stock abutments.

Custom-Made Implant Abutments

Custom abutments, in contrast to stock and UCLA abutments, are recommended for adverse tissue or bone levels relative to the tissue crest because they are pre-milled or cast prior to their placement. This specificity is possible because the abutment is fabricated according to the positioning requirements specific to the patient's needs and dimensions. Further, many options are available for fabricating custom abutments and they can be pre-milled from a variety of materials such as zirconia, titanium, and polyether ketone (PEEK).[1] Consequently, the custom abutment is the most efficient means of restoring an implant crown although it is also the most expensive.

Although there are strength and long-term clinical durability differences between the various materials used for fabricating custom abutments, most are fabricated either from titanium or zirconia. In general, zirconia abutments are preferred when the dental implant is significantly lower than the gingival tissues and, in such situations, extending a metallic abutment to the implant when the collar is metallic may result in a gray shadow from the metallic abutment showing through the gingival tissue. Further, in situations where an all-ceramic based crown is selected for the restoration, a zirconia abutment should provide a superior esthetic outcome than the metallic option.

Although custom abutments are more expensive as they are designed and produced "customized" to the patient, they provide greater accuracy, superior esthetics and a more natural final result. Further, in some cases, the patient's requirements and dental health may not permit the use of stock abutments and custom abutments must be used to achieve optimal outcomes.

The major advantage of custom abutments is that they permit the establishment of both ideal margin placement and an ideal emergence profile. This is shown in Fig. B.2.

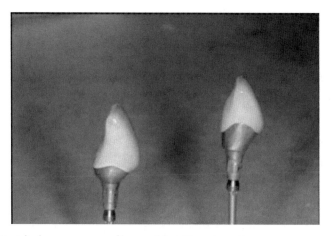

Figure B.2   Ideal emergence profile possible with custom abutments.

An example of the use of custom abutments is shown in the following case.

It is clear from Figs. B.3 – Fig. B.8 that the patient has been provided with good access to the margins so that proper cleaning and maintenance of satisfactory oral hygiene is possible whereas with stock abutments, these clinical requirements may not be possible. It should be noted, however, the major disadvantages of custom abutments are primarily cost and the fact that a cement margin will still exist.

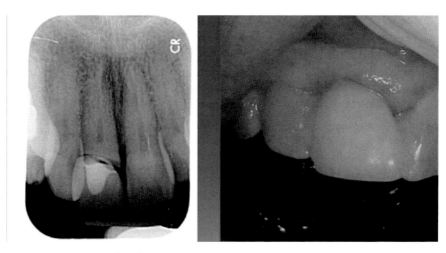

Figure B.3   Fractured tooth #8.

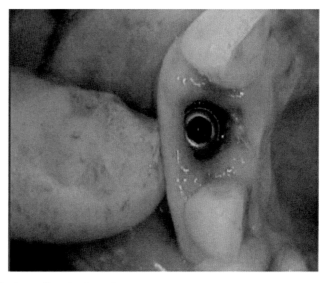

Figure B.4   Immediate implant placement.

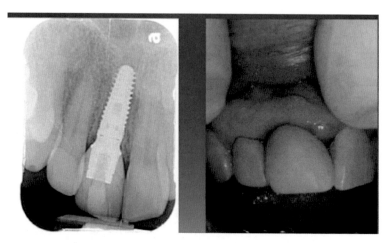

Figure B.5 Immediate temporization.

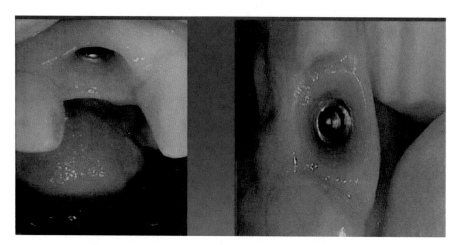

Figure B.6 Soft-tissue profile.

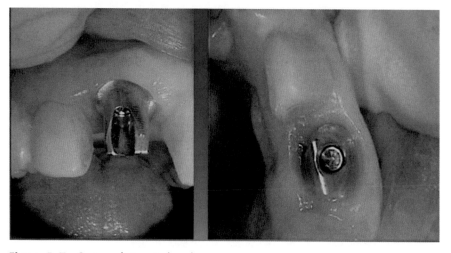

Figure B.7 Custom abutment placed.

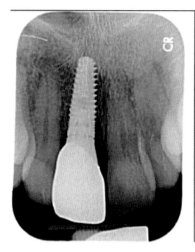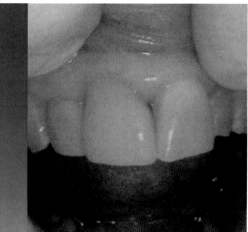

Figure B.8   Final restoration.

Treatment Aspects of Custom Abutments

A prefabricated (stock) abutment is machine-made, seated, and torqued atop the implant. It is then prepared as needed and treated as a conventional post-and-core restorative treatment procedure. Using stock abutments has certain apparent advantages for the patient, notably reduced cost and fewer visits. However, the final outcome may not be as esthetically satisfactory for the patient.

The patient who requires restoration of an implant will present with a healing abutment screwed onto each implant. It is, at this point that, a determination must be made whether to use a custom or prefabricated (stock) abutment. Generally, stock abutments are contra-indicated when:

1. There is insufficient interocclusal space, typically where the abutment might not have sufficient height to retain a crown.
2. The implant requires an angle of correction greater than 15°.
3. The separation between the implant platform and the gingival margin is ≥1 mm greater than the largest commercially available collar height.
4. There is a requirement for splinting three or more implants in a quadrant when parallelism is required. It is generally accepted that when splinting ≥3 implants together in one quadrant, it is very challenging to achieve parallelism.

Following removal of the healing abutment and exposure of the implant restorative platform, a periodontal probe is then used as a guide. In particular, the angle of the implant and its occlusal relationship to the opposing dentition can be assessed visually by situating the shaft of the probe at the center of the implant. If it is decided to use a stock abutment, then the following information is mandatory:

a. The diameter of the implant platform, i.e. whether it is narrow, regular, or wide, although if the implant has been placed by the dentist, then these data should be in the patient treatment notes.

b. The collar or cuff height (i.e., the separation between the implant platform and the gingival margin) at the mesial, distal, buccal, and lingual locations.

c. The interocclusal height (the distance between the implant platform and the opposing dentition), and

d. Whether a straight or angled abutment is needed.

If a custom abutment is to be used, the size of the implant platform is noted and a transfer coping is selected based on an open- or closed-tray design. Thereafter, an impression is taken, and the abutment is fabricated by the lab.

Zirconia Crowns and Abutments

The advent of zirconia in dentistry largely eliminated the design and application limits of all-ceramic restorations as well as the need for porcelain-fused-to-metal (PFM) crowns for high stress areas. In fact, the high strength and fracture toughness of zirconia permits the fabrication of long-span posterior restorations with high accuracy and an excellent success rate. Additionally, the white color of zirconia ensures better reproduction of the required restoration color/tint, especially in the anterior zone. Consequently, given the physical properties of zirconia, its use for the construction of implant abutments and superstructures was a logical step.

Fabricating zirconia implant abutments utilizes state-of-the-art CAD/CAM technology based on the patient's models to produce an individually customized abutment. Further, abutment design in the CAD phase permits accurate positioning and angulation of the zirconia abutment to ensure optimal esthetics. However, fabricating zirconia implant abutments can be complicated by the problem of providing adequate fixation to the implant body. In particular, zirconia is a brittle material and friction between the fixation screw and the internal surface of the ceramic abutment can generate high internal stresses that could lead to unexpected fracture.

This problem has been addressed and probably solved by inserting a friction-fit internal metallic nut that has an external hex to establish proper contact with the implant body. Further, the fixation screw interlocks with the metallic nut during the tightening procedure.

In contrast, fracture risks with zirconia custom abutments and, for example, E.max/zirconia crowns, can be markedly reduced by using a Ti-base. The latter is the internal aspect of a zirconia custom abutment or crown and can be engaging or non-engaging. In much the same way as for zirconia abutments, the Ti-base is scanned and the abutment is designed on a CAD device. Thereafter, the custom abutment, or full contour crown, is then milled on a CAM device before being stained, glazed, and cemented to the Ti-base. It should be noted that the two components, the Ti-base and zirconia/E.max crown, are luted in the lab.

The advantage of titanium custom abutments, compared to Zr-base abutments, is that the fixation screw exerts direct pressure on the abutment which, in turn, has an external or internal hex to provide connection with the implant body. This eliminates any risk of fracture that can potentially occur with zirconia abutments.

Finally, the question of whether the restoration (and, to a degree, the abutment) should be screw- or cement-retained is still under discussion and this subject has been discussed at length in Chapter 13.

Note

1. PEEK or polyether ether ketone is a colorless organic thermoplastic polymer that is used in a variety of engineering applications. It has exceptional mechanical properties and is biocompatible, being FDA approved for food contact.

Appendix C

Bone Graft Materials

It was stated in Chapter 9 that successful placement of implants requires the implant site to have sufficient bone volume of high biologic quality. These requirements, in part, are because the design of the implant necessitates the implant site to possess certain dimensional properties for long-term success and, consequently, bone grafting is often necessary. Other factors necessitating bone grafting include:

- Resorption of the edentulous ridge post-extraction
- Presence of bony defects due to trauma or infection
- The need to place implants in strategic but somewhat unsatisfactory sites for functional and esthetic success.

Both the selection of an appropriate surgical technique and graft material are factors in treatment planning for bone grafting, notably because poor planning or execution can lead to resorption of the graft material or failure to integrate. Another deleterious consequence is the possibility that the lost or removed hard tissue may be replaced by fibrous tissue rather than functional bone. In such cases, osseointegration does not occur and the implant may be doomed to failure.

Bone Grafts in Implant Treatment

The indications and locations for bone grafting are outlined in Table C.1.

After a tooth has been extracted, normal physiological processes result in the loss of 40–60% of the original height and width of the surrounding alveolar bone,

The ADA Practical Guide to Dental Implants, First Edition. Luigi O. Massa and J. Anthony von Fraunhofer.
© 2021 The American Dental Association. Published 2021 by John Wiley & Sons, Inc.

Table C.1 Indications for bone grafting.

1. Alveolar sockets post-extraction
2. Refilling a local bony defect resulting from trauma or infection
3. Refilling a peri-implant defect due to peri-implantitis
4. Vertical augmentation of the mandible and/or maxilla
5. Horizontal augmentation of the mandible and maxilla

the greatest loss occurring within the first two years. This bone loss occurs because the alveolar bundle bone into which the collagen fibers of the periodontium are anchored is dependent on the presence of a tooth and without the tooth, collapse occurs.

Following this loss of alveolar bone, the biological condition of the implant site may adversely affect the proper axial alignment of the implant required for function and esthetics. Thus, minimizing post-extraction alveolar atrophy usually requires the socket to be filled with bone or bone substitute material (BSM), with or without a membrane. These procedures are commonly referred to as "socket preservation" or "ridge preservation" and are designed to:

• Fill the socket
• Preserve the ridge volume
• Promote new bone formation (osteogenesis)
• Avoid the need for later bone/socket augmentation procedures.

Ridge preservation techniques effectively limit horizontal and vertical bone loss following tooth extraction and are far superior in this regard than the healing and bone formation effects found with unsupported blood clotting. Clinical findings indicate that ridge preservation can achieve significant maintenance of ridge width and height and there appears to be little difference in the effectiveness of different graft materials when used for this purpose.

External augmentation procedures on the alveolar ridge are clinically more challenging than the "internal" augmentation procedures (i.e. placing graft materials within the socket), especially in areas like the maxillary sinus.

Interestingly, ridge preservation procedures appear to delay osteogenesis during early healing but, long-term, they significantly reduce ridge atrophy. It has also been found that increasing the width of the alveolar ridge (i.e., horizontal bone augmentation) is more predictable and successful than vertical augmentation and has fewer complications.

Successful Bone Grafting

Following graft placement, bone healing and new bone formation can occur through three physiological processes, namely osteogenesis, osteoinduction, and osteoconduction. For these physiological processes to proceed successfully, the graft site must satisfy certain criteria:

1. Osteoblasts must be present at the site
2. Blood supply at the site must be sufficient for nourishment

3. Soft tissue must not be under tension (or compression)
4. The graft must be stabilized during healing.

Likewise, the graft materials must possess certain properties/characteristics:

a. Osteogenic graft materials must supply viable osteoblasts.
b. Osteoinductive materials should stimulate the differentiation of mesenchymal cells delivered to the site by the blood supply from adjacent bone or periosteum into osteoblasts.
c. Osteoconductive materials should provide a lattice or framework for cell growth and allow osteoblasts from the wound margin to infiltrate the defect and migrate across the graft, thereby stimulating osteoblastic activity within the graft site.

Bone quality at the recipient site determines the type of graft material to be used and a basic rule is that cortical bone is inferior to cancellous bone at the recipient site. This is because cells within cancellous bone provide ≥60% of overall bone healing capacity whereas cells in cortical bone are responsible for only 10% of bone healing. Complicating the issue is that, following tooth extraction, when bone resorption occurs, cancellous bone shrinks relative to cortical bone. Consequently, as the volume of cancellous bone diminishes, there is an associated loss of osteoblasts and other cells. The good thing is that the clinician can use computerized tomography (CT) to indicate the ratio of cancellous to cortical bone at the recipient site prior to surgery and knowledge of this ratio helps in the selection of graft material.

The present consensus with regard to grafting material selection is:

• Predominantly cancellous bone: almost any graft material can be used.
• Mixed cancellous-cortical bone: graft material selection depends upon which type of bone predominates.
• Cortical bone: autograft material is the optimal choice.

Osteoblasis

The graft material properties indicated above are mandatory because only osteoblasts create new bone and the graft matrix must contain, or stimulate proliferation of, osteoblasts to avoid failure of the graft. For osteoblasis to occur, there must be a good blood supply to the graft and surrounding tissue to ensure cell viability and clot formation; the latter functioning as the initial matrix into which cells migrate and then provides anchorage for the osteoblasts.

Graft Stabilization

Any mechanical stress on the graft during the healing process can cause disruption of the fibrin clot and, in particular, movement of the graft will result in fibrous tissue filling the defect instead of bone. Although formation of fibrous tissue is a repair process, it is not, and cannot be, bone regeneration. Accordingly, fixation by GBR (Guided Bone Regeneration) and placement of collagen membranes, titanium mesh or bone screws are recommended in situations where there is a risk of stress-induced graft displacement.

The advantage of GBR is that the grafted site is separated from the surrounding soft tissue, and the GBR membrane isolates the defect from faster-growing tissues like epithelium, fibrous tissue or gingival connective tissue. This allows controlled regeneration of bone. Further, placing bone graft material into the defect prevents collapse of the collagen membrane while functioning as a "place holder" or scaffold for new regenerating bone and as an osteoconductive scaffold for the ingrowth of blood vessels and osteoblasts.

Bone Graft Materials

There are four broad categories of bone graft material, Table C.2, and each has certain advantages and disadvantages.

Table C.2   Bone graft materials.

Graft material	Source
Autograft (autogenous graft)	Hard tissue transferred from one location to another within the same individual.
Allograft (allogenic)	A graft between genetically dissimilar members of the same species, e.g., cadaveric human tissue.
Xenograft	A graft taken from a donor of another species, e.g., bovine or porcine hard tissue.
Alloplast	Inorganic, synthetic, or inert foreign material designed for implantation into tissue.

Autografts

The ideal bone grafting approach is to use the autogenous graft, where hard tissue is transferred from one location to another in the same individual. The autograft is the patient's own bone and, commonly, it is harvested intraorally or from other locations such as the iliac crest or patella plate. It is the ideal bone substitute since it contains living cells and human growth factors and, therefore, has greater osteogenic potential than any other bone substitute as well as an inherent biocompatibility. The vital cells and growth factors within the transferred material provide biological activity so that the grafted material is osteogenic, osteoinductive, and osteoconductive.

It should be noted, however, that the cells in the autogenous bone die within a few days. Thereafter, the block of transferred bone will function as a stable but non-vital slowly resorbable membrane. Allogenic (allograft) bone blocks, functioning as a substitute for autogenous bone (see below), likewise can be used for this base or scaffold purpose, as discussed below. The latter approach eliminates the need for bone harvesting and then sectioning the autogenous bone blocks to particles of the required dimensions.

Despite there being no risk of disease transmission with autogenic grafting, there is always a possibility of pain, infection, and donor site morbidity. Another disadvantage of autogenic grafting is the need for additional surgeries which can increase the complexity of the overall surgical procedure. Further, there is a limited supply of bone available for harvesting, added to which is the risk that bone, once separated from its blood supply, will "die" and this can lead to poor osteoblasis/osteogenesis.

BSMs were developed to overcome the various problems associated with autogenous grafts. BSMs can either replace autogenous bone entirely or expand/extend the autogenous graft. These materials need to be effective for time-delayed procedures, i.e., those performed prior to implant placement, and for simultaneous procedures performed to optimize conditions at the recipient site during implant placement.

Allografts

Allograft materials can be obtained from cadavers or living donors; in the latter case, tissue is typically harvested during hip replacement surgery or similar extensive surgeries. The advantage of allograft materials is that they have the same structure and composition as natural bone but although they are osteoinductive and osteoconductive, they are not osteogenic because they contain no viable osteoblastic cells. Questions have also been asked regarding the risk of transmission of infections such as HIV and hepatitis B and C and, potentially, prions, toxins, systemic disorders and neoplastic tissue. Immunologic responses can occur with allografts although modern processing technologies[1] have virtually eliminated this problem. The good thing is that the processed graft material encourages improved penetration of the surrounding tissues into the graft.

Allograft materials are available either as mineralized cortico/cancellous or demineralized cortical bone granules, and in different granule/particle sizes, usually in the range of 250–1000 μm. Mineralized cortico/cancellous allograft material is a mixture of slower resorbing cortical bone and faster resorbing cancellous bone and requires four to six months for complete turnover. It is commonly used for GBR procedures, typically for wall defects and for socket preservation with time-delayed procedures (Fig. C.1). In contrast, demineralized

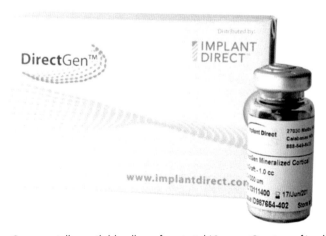

Figure C.1   Commercially-available allograft material (*Source:* Courtesy of Implant Direct).

cortical bone is faster resorbing and there is complete turnover within two to three months. This material is commonly used for "filling the gap" and for socket preservation when earlier implant placement into the prepared site is intended.

The bottom line is that allograft bone blocks and granules are a predictable and effective alternative to the traditional autogenous block for grafting and ridge augmentation. In situations when large areas need to be filled by grafting, a shell of autogenous bone is often used as a "biologic" base or scaffold to create the necessary space for the incorporation of the granulated bone graft material. The bone cells in the autogenous bone die within a few days and then the bone plate functions as a stable, non-vital, slowly resorbable barrier. Allogenic bone blocks can also be used as a substitute for autogenous bone for this shell technique, which avoids the need for harvesting and splitting of the autogenous bone blocks. Histologic studies indicate that there are no differences in the final stage of incorporation between autografts and allografts.

A convenient allograft material is DirectGen™ Dental DBM Putty which is comprised 100% of demineralized bone. The putty consistency simplifies handling and molding, particularly for GBR and grafting around implants while possessing maximized allograft content.

Xenografts

Xenogeneic materials are those derived from other organisms, principally from bovine or porcine sources. Because animal bones comprise natural and slightly porous hydroxyapatite, these xenografts are osteoconductive and available in a range of particle sizes which, when placed in position, will maintain long-term volume stability.

Demineralized bovine bone (e.g., DirectOss™) has long been used for xenografts. The harvested material is deproteinized by heating to eliminate any risk of allergic reactions and disease transmission. The final thermal product, basically a biologically-derived hydroxyapatite quasi-ceramic, has a structure similar to that of human bone. In particular, the trabecular bone architecture with its interconnecting pores provides near-optimal conditions for ingrowth of new vascularity from the surrounding tissues. The net result is guided osseointegration rather than rapid resorption which, in turn, leads to good stability of the volume of graft material with the formation of new bone on the surface and within the highly structured bovine bone.

Bovine bone is extremely slow resorbing and, when implanted, particles may still be present at 24 months following placement. However, when a longer turnover is required, this material is sometimes mixed with mineralized cortico/cancellous particles in GBR.

Another xenografting option is the use of bovine collagen, e.g., Foundation®. This approach utilizes a mixture of untreated collagen, which acts as a scaffold, and heat-denatured collagen, which stimulates growth. When the mixture is freeze-dried and cross-linked by heat, it is then processed into a sponge block and formed into a conical shape for easy placement into the extraction socket. Clinical studies show stimulation of new bone occurs at an accelerated pace.

Because the xenoplastic material is synthetically produced, there is no risk of disease transmission.

Membranes

Membranes are flexible, semipermeable xenograft materials placed in the area of the dental implant, bone defect or ridge reconstruction to aid in wound healing [1]. They are designed to conform to the contours of the defect site and allow nutrient exchange while providing a barrier to prevent epithelial downgrowth. Two types of membrane exist; resorbable and non-resorbable.

Resorbable membranes, e.g., Kontour™ and Sustain Kontour, are highly biocompatible materials fabricated from a nonfriable, conformable matrix engineered from highly purified type I collagen derived from porcine tendon. Such membranes resorb within four to six months and are used for GBR. They tend to be less suitable in sites where there is continuing exposure to oral cavity.

In contrast, non-resorbable membranes are fabricated from high-density polytetrafluoroethylene (PTFE), e.g., Cytoplast™ TXT-200, which are designed for guided tissue regeneration membrane for extraction site grafting and augmentation procedures. They are particularly suitable in situations where exposure to the oral cavity is common. They usually have a microtextured surface that increases the surface area for enhanced soft-tissue attachment but are resistant to bacterial invasion because of their nanoscale porosity. The result of this approach to membrane design is that the membrane can be left exposed in the mouth without complications.

Both resorbable and non-resorbable membranes are clinically very useful. Resorbable materials have the great advantage that they do not need to be retrieved at a later date, but they are more costly although more convenient than non-resorbable membranes which must be retrieved at a later date.

Alloplasts

The most common alloplastic materials are calcium phosphate-based ceramics such as hydroxyapatite (HA) and tricalcium phosphate (TCP). One material, GUIDOR® easy-graft, is marketed as a homogenous moldable mass, which is applied directly from the syringe and is available as a HA-TCP (65 : 35 and 55 : 45 ratio of HA to TCP) mixture and TCP-only formulations.

When pressed into the defect, compaction of the GUIDOR easy-graft forces permeation of blood between the granules and the material hardens quickly to form a scaffold of interconnected granules that conforms to the morphology of the defect. Larger defects may typically require a second and immediate application of additional material to ensure adequate defect filling. The hardened material is slightly porous with a structure analogous to that of bone and, consequently, it can help stabilize the fibrin clot essential in the initial stages of healing.

Calcium phosphate alloplastic materials are bioactive and resorbable, both characteristics enabling the attachment and proliferation of bone cells. Initially, they become integrated into the surrounding bone matrix and then undergo a gradual remodeling and degradation. However, whereas both HA and TCP have no immunogenic or toxic effects and exhibit blood biocompatibility and osteo-conductivity, they have no osteogenic or osteoinductive properties. Consequently, neither material can provide immediate structural support.

The principle behind using an HA-TCP combination as a bone regeneration material is that the alloplast should resorb at the same rate as the formation of new bone. Clinically, the HA portion resorbs slowly and remains integrated in the newly formed bone whereas the TCP resorbs and is replaced by new bone which becomes embedded in the remaining HA component to create a stable scaffold. The very slow HA resorption ensures the long-term volume stability of the graft and provides a good substrate for the proliferation of osteoinductive growth factors and osteogenic cells.

Bioactive glass is another alloplastic bone substitute which is used extensively in dentistry and orthopedic surgery because of its greater bioactivity compared to that of TCP and HA. Bioactive glass has the ability to promote natural bone regeneration through sustained ion release. After placement, it will react with blood and bond to bone, where it releases silica and other mineral ions which, in turn, stimulate osteoblast differentiation and proliferation. Over the long term, bioactive glass will be completely resorbed and be replaced by bone. Research indicates that when bioactive glass is mixed with autogenous bone graft material, the rate of natural bone regeneration appears to double.

Conclusions

The consensus is that the survival rates of implants placed into grafted areas are comparable with those of implants placed into "pristine" bone. However, the bone quality at the recipient site is a key determinant of the type of graft material to be used, with cortical bone being inferior to cancellous bone at the implant site.

Ridge preservation techniques are effective in limiting horizontal and vertical bone loss post-extraction compared to healing by blood clot alone in that they will maintain ridge width and height. Clinical studies indicate that most graft materials are effective for this purpose with only small differences between them depending, of course, on the bone quality at the implant site. However, it should be noted that autogenous onlay bone grafting procedures are effective with predictable outcomes when correcting severely resorbed edentulous ridges, but survival rates may be slightly lower than those of implants placed in pristine bone. It should also be noted that, at this time, there is a paucity of data on the longevity of preserved ridges and the survival rates of the implants placed in these areas.

Finally, regardless of the graft material, poor blood supply, trauma or extensive surgery and, particularly, thermal or frictional damage during site preparation, will usually adversely affect the implant prognosis. Further, diseases that affect bone metabolism, e.g., uncontrolled diabetes, head/neck irradiation and bisphosphonates likewise adversely affect implant prognoses. It should also be mentioned that smokers and tobacco users generally experience a higher prevalence of complications with implants.

Note

1. Briefly, processing of allograft tissue involves ultrasonic cleaning to remove blood and soft tissue as well as fat from the cancellous bone structure. Thereafter, chemical treatment denatures non-collagen proteins, destroys bacteria and inactivates viruses whereas oxidation denatures any retained soluble proteins and eliminates potential immunogenicity. Structural integrity is preserved by dehydration and sterility is ensured through gamma irradiation.

Reference

Elgali, I., Omar, O., Dahlin, C., and Thomsen, P. (2017). Guided bone regeneration: materials and biological mechanisms revisited. *Eur. J. Oral Sci.* 125: 315–337.

Index

Page numbers in *italic* indicate tables.

The ADA Practical Guide to Dental Implants, First Edition. Luigi O. Massa and J. Anthony von Fraunhofer.
© 2021 The American Dental Association. Published 2021 by John Wiley & Sons, Inc.

Made in United States
Orlando, FL
09 June 2024

47681128R00108